fit for life

A THINNER
YOU

Credits:

Art Director: Peter Bridgewater
Editorial Consultants: Maria Pal/Clark Robinson Ltd

Picture credits:

key: b = below; i = inset; l = left

The author and publishers have made every effort to identify the
copyright owners of the photographs; they apologize for any
omissions and wish to thank the following:

Clive Boden, 13, 20–21, 25, 29, 39, 78–79, 82, 83; David Burch,
71, 24, 26, 28, 85; Sheila Buff, 74; Paul Forrester, 19, 76; David
Gallant, 53; John Heseltine, 21i, 33, 34–35, 41, 43, 47, 48, 49, 50,
63, 65b, 66–67, 73b,·87, 88, 89; Hing/Norton, 80, 81; Western NC
Farmers' Market, 8–9; Trevor Wood, 16; Trevor Wood/Michael
Bull, 52.

fit for life

A THINNER
YOU

ABBOT NEIL SOLOMON

Gallery Books
an imprint of W.H. Smith Publishers, Inc.
112 Madison Avenue, New York
New York 10016

A QUARTO BOOK

This edition published in 1990 by Gallery Books,
an imprint of W.H. Smith Publishers, Inc.,
112, Madison Avenue, New York, New York 10016

Gallery Books are available for bulk purchase for
sales promotions and premium use. For details write or
telephone the Manager of Special Sales, W.H. Smith
Publishers Inc., 112 Madison Avenue, New York, New
York 10016. (212) 532-6600.

ISBN 0-8317-3896-0

The information and recommendations contained in this book
are intended to complement, not substitute for, the advice of
your own physician. Before starting any medical treatment,
exercise program or diet, consult your physician. Information is
given without any guarantees on the part of the author and
publisher, and they cannot be held responsible for the contents
of this book.

► CONTENTS

SENSIBLE WEIGHT LOSS

Any sensible weight-loss program should combine a diet and an energy-efficient exercise regimen. Changing your eating and exercise habits requires a constant and conscious effort. Eating habits are ingrained from childhood and carry various emotional attachments. For example, many of us eat to overcome depression. Few people eat in response to hunger alone.

Do not underestimate the importance of making changes in the food you eat. The general level of chronic poor health is so widespread that it has become accepted, and a lot of people have forgotten what it is like to really feel well and active. Many of the foods we eat tend to be counterproductive to energy. Full of additives, overprocessed, or lacking nutrients, some of these foods discourage an active lifestyle, which leads to weight gain and lethargy.

Changing to a whole-food way of eating, with lots of fresh food, can lead to a radical and speedy improvement in your health and vitality, and this will benefit other areas of your life. Foods that in the past were thought of as luxuries, but are now commonplace,

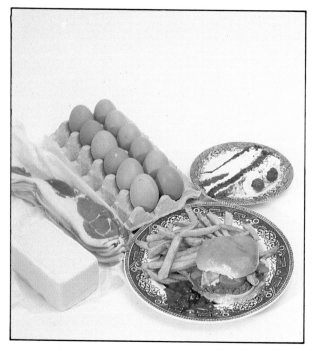

Giving up old eating habits isn't a simple step, but one that will bring immediate rewards. A good way to start is by making a list (right) of the type of changes you want to make in your diet. Foods high in cholesterol, such as dairy products and fatty meats (left) should be given a low priority, whereas fresh fruit and vegetables should play a prominent role.

such as cream, pastries, and lavish helpings of meat, should be once more limited to special occasions. Scientific studies have shown that the best diet is one based on whole grains, vegetables, and fruit, with small amounts of meat and dairy products as a complement to a meal, rather than its basis. The central idea is to eat fresh, whole foods and avoid or restrict the intake of fats, refined sugar, white 'flour, red meat, and processed foods, containing chemical additives.

To lose weight you should not go on a diet that is just low in calories, because studies have shown that the body's metabolism slows down in response to a cutback in food quantity. Low-calorie diets tend to make you sluggish and lazy, reducing your desire to burn up fat-causing foods with exercise.

Any sensible diet must include an exercise routine. The trick is to make the exercise enjoyable enough that you like to do it. Don't start out with a routine so complicated or difficult that you look for ways to avoid it. Before beginning any diet or exercise program, consult you doctor.

Combining your new exercise workout with a new approach to eating will lead to a thinner you!

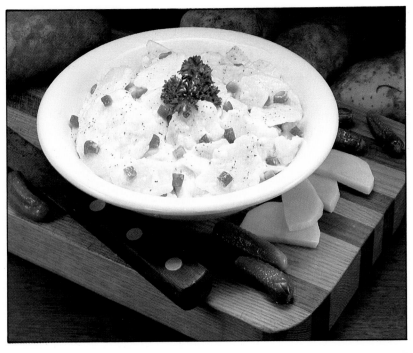

PROCESSED FOOD

Increasingly, the food-manufacturing industries are processing, refining, preserving, and packaging more and more foods. In the process they have created food that is energy-dense but nutritionally poor. These packaged foods are high in calories and low in goodness.

When we talk of a food being calorie-dense, we mean it is high in calories. A calorie is a measure of the amount of energy or heat given off by the food when metabolized by the body. The body needs six nutrients: water, proteins, fats, carbohydrates, vitamins, and minerals.

In processed, manufactured food, the sugar, fats, and white flour have all been refined and treated to remove the perishable substances. It is these living parts, such as the wheat germ in wheat, that contain the goodness. After their removal what is left is a

"Whole-foods" are foods that have not been processed in any way, and fresh fruit and vegetables are among the very best examples. For many people, discovering the variety and versatility of the produce available is an eye-opener. It also makes shopping a visual delight.

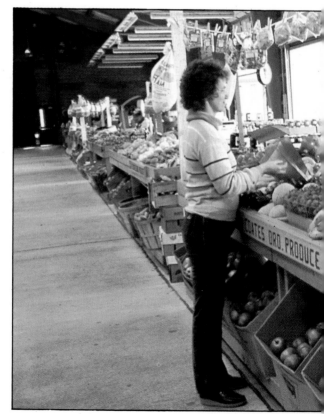

product that is pliable, durable, bland, versatile, and consistent — all ideal qualities for processing foods by machines and keeping the packages for great lengths of time on supermarket shelves. Chemical additives and coloring agents are added to ensure that the products have standard flavor, long life, and are bright enough to attract the eye. But refined sugar, refined flour, and commercial fats contain nothing but calories!

Although manufactured food is quicker and easier to put on your table, these new foods are thought to lead to an increase in chronic diseases. Science has shown that many degenerative diseases are caused not necessarily by old age, but by our lifestyle and particularly by the food we eat. The single major cause of heart disease, many respiratory ailments and digestive diseases, and 35 percent of cancer, is now thought to be our diet — high in refined flour and sugar, fat, red meat, and alcohol, but low in vegetables, fruit, whole grains, cereals, and beans.

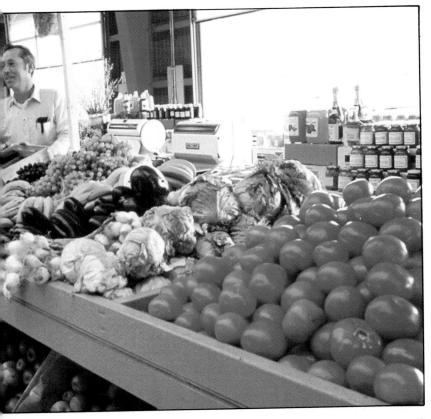

ADDITIVES

Currently there are over 3,000 food additives in use. Besides pesticides, fungicides, and anti-oxidants, there are many more substances used to make food look plumper or give it a brighter color.

These chemical additives can cause a wide range of adverse effects, but while medicines must be carefully tested, before they can be offered, many additives are not. It can cost up to a million dollars to test an additive, and in any case it is difficult to test them conclusively, since chemicals added to food are not consumed in prescribed doses as drugs are. What may be a safe intake in small portions of food may become hazardous if larger quantities are eaten. There is also the chance that if you mix two harmless chemicals together you may end up with a harmful concoction.

Chemical additives have been cited as a cause in the great rise of some cancers in the last few decades. Many of the additives we eat are not excreted but are stored in our body fat, liver, and other organs. Children are especially vulnerable; they excrete only 50 percent of the chemical additives they take in, whereas adults eliminate up to 90 percent.

Some additives are necessary to preserve processed foods, such as sodium nitrate used in ham to protect us from botulism. Vitamin C is used as an anti-oxidant and may have beneficial effects.

An average loaf of commercial bread contains about 34 additives, among them chlorine gas, used as an oxidizing agent to make the flour stiffer and easier to bake. This increases the amount of bread that can be made and in turn means a lower cost for the consumer.

Unless you grow your own food, it is becoming increasingly difficult to keep away from chemical additives. However, if you can learn to be selective, you can diminish the amount of additives in your new diet. Since it has been shown that sodium nitrate in bacon, for example, releases cancer-causing nitrites when cooked, a wise decision would be to give up processed pork.

Since livestock, fruits, and vegetables are treated with pesticides, we are all likely to have some of these chemicals stored in our body fat. This is a major reason many people avoid meat; it also shows the need to wash fruit and vegetables well.

The average processed white loaf contains about 34 additives, among them chlorine gas, and very little fiber. *Opt instead for brown bread (opposite), made from wholemeal or wholewheat flour.*

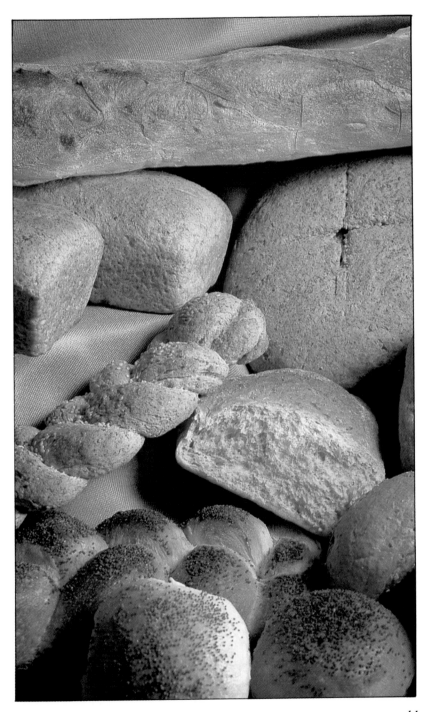

NUTRITION PROPERTIES

Eating healthy is simple; there are no complicated diets, no tortuous rules or expensive shopping lists. Wholesome, nourishing food is varied, interesting and tasty. And a balanced, nutrition-oriented diet will help you slim down by making you conscious of what you eat!

The benefits of adopting simpler, fresher ways of eating are felt by most people immediately. The body responds quickly to the lightening of the load placed on the digestive system, experiencing an increase in long-term energy from the slow-burning carbohydrates and enjoying the healthy, cleansing effects of lots of fresh fruits and vegetables.

The simple process of moving away from the quick snacks of sugar- and fat-laden foods will have a beneficial effect on your ability to cope with the demands of a busy life. Your blood sugar levels will even out, ridding you of those undermining mood swings.

Many people also find that they lose weight easily and naturally. If you need to lose weight, then your body, given the assistance of a nutritionally balanced diet, will lose as fast or as slowly as it is ready.

It is much harder to overeat whole, nourishing foods. Your body's signals telling you to "stop eating" respond better on unrefined foods.

Following the eating plan in this book is one of the better cures for people who gorge, and for those of us with insatiable cravings. The rewards of eating fresh whole foods and a high proportion of fresh fruit and vegetables are not just an absence of illness or the curing of certain diseases. Eating well is enjoyable as well as a vital part of positive health.

What we outline in this book is a sensible way to adjust your diet toward healthy foods. By combining the required basics with a few interesting complements and treats, you'll be on your way to a thinner you!

Remember that each person's metabolism is as individual as a set of fingerprints. No two people have the same nutritional requirements; what is nearly indigestible for one person may help another to thrive. Make the necessary adjustments to suit your own needs. By adopting some of these suggestions and realigning your food priorities according to the way you feel, you'll begin leading a healthier life!

Raw vegetables, *attractively and tastily made up into salads that combine a number of different ingredients should make a regular appearance in your diet. Packed with vitamins and minerals, with none lost through cooking, salads provide you with masses of energy without affecting your waistline.*

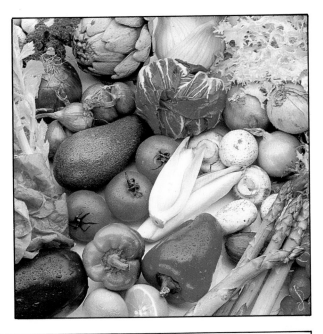

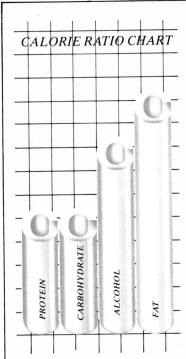

CALORIE RATIO CHART

PROTEIN

CARBOHYDRATE

ALCOHOL

FAT

Becoming aware of the calorie content *of particular types of foods will enable you to regulate your diet for optimum health. Alcohol, for example, is one of the most concentrated sources of energy, and if you are in the habit of drinking regularly, after work, for example, you should make allowance for this when reviewing your calorie intake. Not all high-calorie foods should necessarily be avoided — they may supply valuable nutrients, and everyone needs a certain amount of fat in the diet — the important thing is to devise an eating plan that incorporates protein, carbohydrates and fat in healthy proportions.*

ENERGY BALANCE AND WEIGHT

If the input of energy from your food exceeds the use of energy through your physical activity, the difference is stored in your body as fat. Many people accept that they will put on weight as they grow older. This is not a natural or inevitable process. Ideally, a person's weight should remain constant after reaching adulthood. There is only one way to achieve this — to balance the number of calories eaten to the number of calories used!

About 20 tons of food are eaten during an average lifetime. With that figure in mind, you can see that even a small energy imbalance can have an extraordinary cumulative effect. An extra 50 calories a day, whether from an extra pat of butter or from driving to a nearby store instead of walking, can result in a substantial weight gain in just a few years.

To lose weight rapidly, most people need to eat at least 1,000 calories less than their average daily expenditure of energy. If this is done, the body has to use (and reduce) its stores of fat to make up the deficit. A diet that combines exercise with calorie reduction is the most sensible way to get the slimming energy balance!

Individual energy requirements vary widely. Some people use over three times more energy each day than others. Most of these differences are due to the varying amounts of energy needed for different physical activities. Other factors are body weight, age, and, to a lesser extent, climate. The speed with which energy is used by the body — the metabolic rate — also varies from person to person.

Without a lengthy series of tests, it is impossible to predict exactly how much energy an individual person needs over an average day or even for a specific activity. However, the average energy expended in a number of given routines show the wide disparity in calorie burning. An average man uses about 2,380 calories a day; 524 during eight hours of sleep; 856 while at work in an office job; and 1,000 in a variety of activities such as cleaning and watching television. Obviously, the more strenuous the activity, the more calories are burned.

The energy used in various common daily activities by a man of 140 pounds and a woman of 120 pounds.

Activities	KJs	4.1868	8.3736	12.5604	16.7472	20.934	25.1208	29.3076	33.4944
Asleep in bed									
Sitting quietly									
Standing quietly									
Cooking									
Light cleaning									
Moderate cleaning (polishing)									
Walking at 3mph									
Sedentary work									
office									
driving									
Light industry									
garage repairs, laundry work									
electrical work									
Recreations									
seated (knitting)									
light (golf, sailing)									
moderate (dancing, riding)									
heavy (athletics, football)									

Men   Women   Approximate amount of energy used on average each minute

EXERCISE TO CURE FOOD ADDICTIONS

While dieting is essentially a negative activity that is self-denying and restrictive, exercise is a positive discipline. When you take up a form of exercise you commit yourself to doing something *for* your body, instead of keeping something away from it!

As well as helping to maintain weight, exercise helps counter cravings for processed foods, and establishes a healthy, "real" appetite for nourishing foods. In the same way, many people who smoke find that after taking up exercise they lose their desire, sometimes quickly, for nicotine.

The physiological reasons for this are simple. Regular exercise stimulates the release of norepinephrine into the bloodsteam. This hormone, together with adrenaline, is released from the adrenal glands, just above the kidneys, in response to activity and stress. The two hormones work to release sugar into the blood, preparing the body for action. Norepinephrine is the hormone that responds to pleasurable stress, like sex and physical exercise, and active emotions, like anger and competitiveness. The increase in exercise causes the hormones to be released, allowing the body to respond "naturally" to the stress of making you reach for the "calming" cigarette!

These physiological reactions, which take place during exercise, combine with the increased blood circulation and general enjoy-

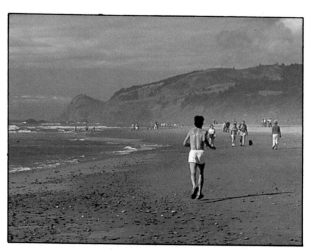

The benefits of exercise are so numerous, and the ill-effects of a sedentary lifestyle so well-established, that there is no good excuse for not taking up regular physical activity of some kind.

ment of movement to help replace harmful addictions with natural and beneficial physical improvements.

Research studies into the benefits of exercise show it to be remarkably effective in combating depression, anxiety, and other negative and self-destructive emotions. Since many people respond to these anxieties and depressions by munching on junk food or smoking cigarettes, a steady, enjoyable exercise plan not only leads to a thinner you, but also to a healthier and happier you!

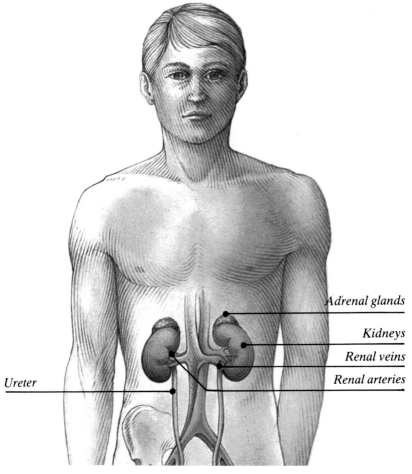

Adrenal glands

Kidneys

Renal veins

Renal arteries

Ureter

Regular exercise stimulates the release by the adrenal glands of norepinephrine and adrenaline into the bloodstream. These two hormones allow the body to respond "naturally" to the types of stress that tends to provoke harmful addictions — whether they are to junk food or cigarettes.

THE SECRET WORKOUT

Many of us break out into a sweat just thinking about exercise. Since sweating alone isn't enough to burn off some of those calories, there are ways to exercise just by increasing certain activities of your normal routine. Here are some excellent secret workouts:

THE ISOMETRIC DESK WORKOUT
It's the middle of the day, and you're feeling a little tense and need to relax. Here's a secret exercise that not only helps you relax but also tightens your biceps and abdomen. Push your chair about eight inches away from the desk. Placing both your palms face up under the desk, sit erect in the chair and hold in your stomach. Then gently press up with your palms against the desk. Release. Repeat five times.

THE WALK DON'T RUN WORKOUT
Many of us lack the time or desire to run a few miles every day. But we all have to walk at some point, so take advantage of that and burn off some calories. The next time you go for a walk, try moving at a brisker pace. Also, move your arms back and forth, flexing them as you do. The faster you walk, the more calories you'll burn. By keeping the arms moving, you'll also be strengthening your upper body.

THE TELEVISION TUCK
Who said watching television is bad for your health? Next time you're glued to the set, grab hold of the sides of the chair and extend one leg toward the screen. Hold it in place for a few seconds while you hold in your stomach. Then put the foot down and repeat the exercise with the other leg. By doing this a few times, you'll tighten up your legs and stomach.

THE ROCK-AND-ROLL WORKOUT
Since so many of us are into aerobic workouts to tighten the muscles and strengthen the heart, what better, more sociable place to do it than in a dance club? Just get out on the floor, join the crowd, and dance away. You won't even realize that all that hopping, leaping, and shaking is an aerobic workout.

At work (opposite), exercise biceps by pressing your palms up beneath your desktop. Keep your back straight and hold your stomach in.

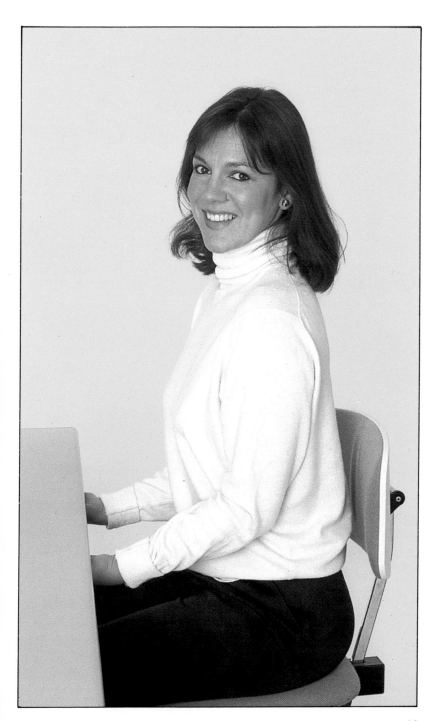

HEALTHY BASICS

Lettuces and green leafy vegetables are healthy, versatile and various. The basic rules for making good salads are to select fine fresh produce and to prepare and eat it as soon as possible. Low-calorie dressings and extra ingredients including nuts, bean sprouts and tofu can be used to introduce endless variety and create nutritious, delicious and attractive salads. Experiment with some of the more unusual lettuces and salad greens such as:

● mignonette lettuce which is similar to a romaine lettuce in form, with dark green or red-tinged outer leaves and a good flavor.

● choy sum which is recognizable by its small yellow flowers and

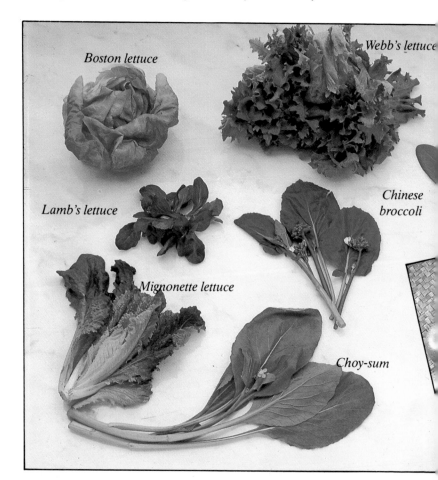

Boston lettuce

Webb's lettuce

Lamb's lettuce

Chinese broccoli

Mignonette lettuce

Choy-sum

grooved stems and its mild cabbage flavor.

● Chinese broccoli with its more pronounced cabbage flavor. The stalks of this green are particularly delicious.

● sorrel with its lemony, sour, tart flavor. Sorrel is grown commercially and is also found in the wild. For salads it is best to use the tender young leaves.

● cress with its slightly sharp taste.

● Webb's lettuce which is a widely cultivated variety. It has curly leaves and is crisper than the soft-leaved Boston lettuce.

● Boston lettuce which has a subtle, sweet, buttery flavor. It is an excellent component in any salad and takes dressings well.

● Lamb's lettuce which is characterized by its tangy taste. it does not travel well so it is usually available only near where it grown or picked.

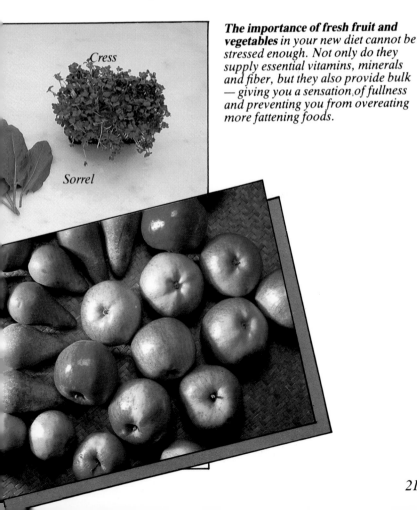

Cress

Sorrel

The importance of fresh fruit and vegetables in your new diet cannot be stressed enough. Not only do they supply essential vitamins, minerals and fiber, but they also provide bulk — giving you a sensation of fullness and preventing you from overeating more fattening foods.

STAYING THIN

The chart here shows the ideal weights for men and women, according to their heights and builds. Once these weights have been achieved, you can begin to eat more high-energy foods, such as chocolates and cheese, provided you keep close tabs on your weight. Even then you must eat sensible, well-balanced foods to stay slim.

A good way to ensure that you keep your weight at the ideal level is to exercise. Exercising to stay slim allows you to eat nourishing, delicious foods and still keep your tummy from slipping over your waist! Since many overweight people eat too much and exercise too little, they often have psychological problems maintaining their new, thinner figures after fighting to get the weight down. It was such a chore to knock off those pounds, that some people feel the need for a reward — like a thick slab of layer cake with a scoop of ice cream. Soon the rewards pile up, along with the calories, and before you can say cheesecake, you're right back where you started.

To avoid this syndrome, get into the enjoyable exercise habit. Choose exercises that are fun to do. When previously nonactive people start a more active lifestyle, they quickly realize their tolerance for a physical effort is limited. At the beginning, exercise quite literally shakes everything up and causes varying degrees of physical discomfort. Your muscles ache and your back hurts, and you tend to ease up on the exercises. Don't! Try resting for a day or so and then get back into your routine. Gradually the aches and pains will disappear and you'll begin to see the benefits of your workout. In the beginning, you'll be running to the mirror to see the "new you," only to see the same layers of flab staring back at you. Losing weight and getting into shape takes time. Keep at it and remember that the hard work will eventually pay off. Soon you'll be digging around the dark recesses of your closet, looking for clothes that haven't fit you in years.

If you need an incentive, cut out a picture of a new outfit from a magazine and tape it to your refrigerator door. That new dress or suit should be your reward, not a chocolate layer cake!

Take into account your build when calculating your desirable weight from a chart (right). Weigh yourself preferably at the same time of day, wearing the same amount of clothing. Standing on the scale once a week, rather than every day, gives a more accurate measure of weight loss.

Height		Small frame	Medium frame	Large frame
Desirable Weights for Men and Women Aged 25 and Over (in pounds, in indoor clothing)				
Men				
Feet	Inches			
5	2	112–120	118–129	126–141
5	3	115–123	121–133	129–144
5	4	118–126	124–136	132–148
5	5	121–129	127–139	135–152
5	6	124–133	130–143	138–156
5	7	128–137	134–147	142–161
5	8	132–141	138–152	147–166
5	9	136–145	142–156	151–170
5	10	140–150	146–160	155–174
5	11	144–154	150–165	159–179
6	0	148–158	154–170	164–184
6	1	152–162	158–175	168–189
6	2	156–167	162–180	173–194
6	3	160–171	167–185	178–199
6	4	164–175	172–190	182–204
Women				
4	10	92–98	96–107	104–119
4	11	94–101	98–110	106–122
5	0	96–104	101–113	109–125
5	1	99–107	104–116	112–128
5	2	102–110	107–119	115–131
5	3	105–113	110–122	118–134
5	4	108–116	113–126	121–138
5	5	111–119	116–130	125–142
5	6	114–123	120–135	129–146
5	7	118–127	124–139	133–150
5	8	122–131	128–143	137–154
5	9	126–135	132–147	141–158
5	10	130–140	136–151	145–163
5	11	134–144	140–155	149–168
6	0	138–148	144–159	153–173

Source: U.S. Public Health Service

THE BASICS

Most people when they hear the term basic food think of sizzling steaks with mashed potatoes and gravy. They might as well be strapping those relatively unhealthy weight-producing foods directly to their waists! In our nutritionally oriented diet, basic foods are items like salads and whole-grain products. These are the basics because besides being low in fats and calories, they provide a good foundation for your healthy meals.

Make sure that a wide range of fruits and vegetables together with beans and cereals forms the basis of your new diet. These foods are the healthiest to eat — they guarantee a low intake of fats and calories, while providing lots of fiber. Since your family may not be accustomed to eating salads or vegetables as a "main course," your goal is to be creative. By beginning to introduce salads garnished with items from the treats and complements, you can devise some tasty alternatives to your old, traditional, unhealthy meals.

Always make sure that the food is fresh and, if possible, organically grown. Organically grown food tends to be lower in chemical additives than processed items. Try to eat as much raw food as

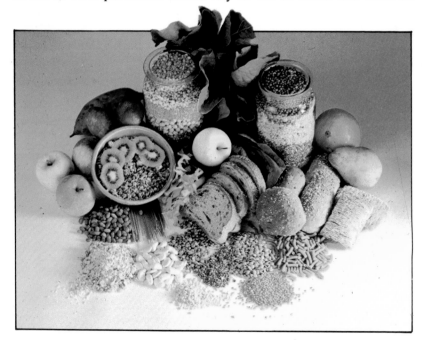

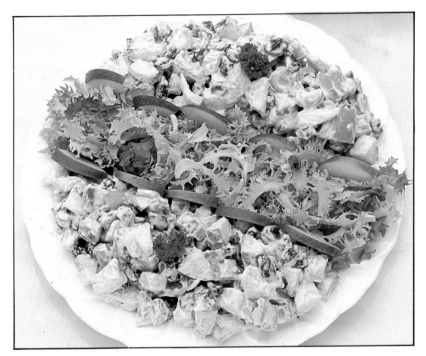

Ideally, treat yourself and your family to a salad once a day. The scope for experiment and variation is endless and the preparation quick and easy. Rather than always making lettuce your salad staple, go for a combination of roots, tubors and leafy vegetables.

possible, at least one salad a day. There are so many quick and easy variations of salad — celery, chopped apples, and raisins, for example — that you should not be stuck for inspiration. When selecting your vegetables choose a wide variety, including roots, tubers, and leafy greens. The dark, leafy, green vegetables provide a rich source of minerals such as iron.

Another basic item is dried beans. A high source of protein, dried beans can be used in tasty combinations in salads, casseroles, and chili. Use them to create dishes of chili con carne, lentil or minestrone soup, and even hummus, a wonderfully tasty Middle Eastern dish made from chickpeas.

The last basic ingredient to your nutritionally sound diet is the cereal group. Whole-wheat products, rye, oats, barley, brown rice and even porridge provide low-fat, high-protein content to your meal. In addition, the cereal group gives your body added fiber, which has been shown to be an excellent deterrent to certain forms of cancer.

THE COMPLEMENTS

If you want to start getting compliments, you have to start eating complements. Complements are the foods that when added to your basics, provide additional nourishment and taste to your new diet. Seeds, nuts, eggs, milk, yogurt, and fish are excellent items as a complement to the basics.

Unlike the basics, which are pretty much totally healthful, the complements have to be somewhat rationed. Eggs, for example are very high in cholesterol and quite rich. They should be eaten less often than other complements — two or three times a week is ideal. Milk should be of the low-fat variety to keep the fat content of your diet under control.

Nature concentrates goodness in the reproductive parts of all creatures. That is why seeds, nuts, and eggs when added to the basics, such as cereal and salads, provide excellent sources of protein and other nutrients.

Sprouted grains and seeds greatly increase their vitamin content as they grow, also becoming an even better source of protein.

Nuts, eggs and dairy produce are useful additions to the basic components of your diet, but should be eaten sparingly because of their high fat and cholesterol levels. Skimmed milk and low-fat cheese are now generally available and can be used as healthier alternatives.

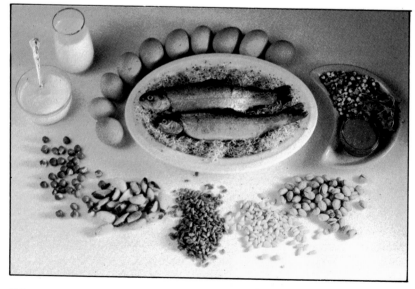

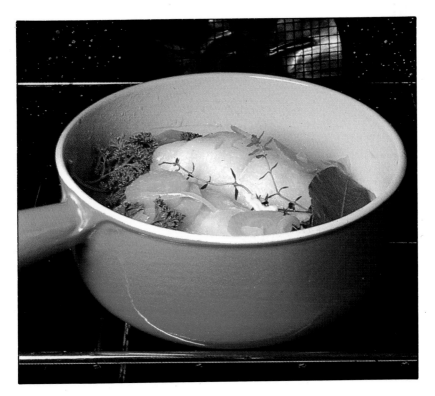

Fish *provides low-fat protein and essential minerals and oils.*

Sprouts should be eaten raw and fresh, for cooking destroys much of their value.

Fish provides another good source of animal protein and essential minerals and oils. Fish roe, like other eggs, are concentrated sources of nourishment. Fish should be served broiled, baked, or poached, seasoned with lemon and herbs not heavy sauces. It provides a low-fat protein and is delicious when cooked with vegetables in stews or curries. Research indicates that fish protein may have a protective effect against certain forms of heart disease.

Low-fat milk and live yogurt are two more excellent sources of protein and other nutrients. Yogurt, delicious in sweet dishes or eaten on its own, makes a good substitute for cream, since it is low in calories and fat and high in protein. Easily assimilated by the body, live yogurt encourages the growth of intestinal bacteria called flora, which aid digestion. Flora are destroyed by highly acid foods (like coffee, tea, sugar, and meat), by antibiotics, alcohol, and other drugs.

THE TREATS

When most people hear the word treat, they immediately think of ice cream, cake, and candy. But the treats we are talking about are foods like cottage cheese, poultry, and red meat. They are considered treats because they should be eaten sparingly.

Meat, poultry, cheese, and other dairy products form the fundamentals of the group we call treats. None of these is essential to health, and they are all relatively expensive. Rich in saturated fat, they are a burden to the digestion, the metabolism, the circulation, and the kidneys. Since they come at the end of the food chain (from seed, to plant, to animal, to manufacturer, to consumer) they are also likely to retain many of the chemicals used in their manufacture and processing. You can still enjoy them, provided you eat them only now and then. By eating a varied and imaginative whole food diet, though, you will probably find that your appetite for these treats actually decreases.

Poultry is preferable to red meat, which you should eat only in minimal quantities. Instead of serving a whole steak or hamburgers, use the meat in smaller quantities — in a pasta sauce, for example.

Another treat item includes whole-wheat baked goods. Tradi-

The treats, *foods such as red meat, fatty poultry, cakes and biscuits need not be avoided altogether, but are best eaten only infrequently.*

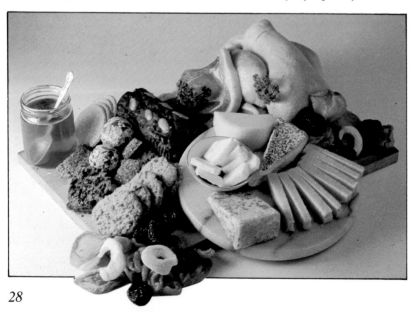

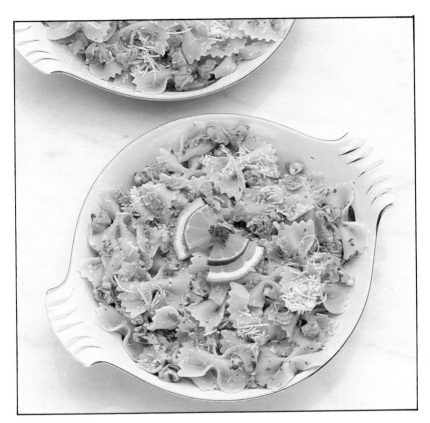

Pasta and clams — *an ideal combination of carbohydrate and protein.*

tional cakes, cookies, and pastry are all high in fat and sugar. The sugar content of your occasional whole food treats should come instead from dried fruit, or substitute honey or molasses, which are just as sweet as sugar. Honey and molasses also contain some traces of essential elements, minerals, and vitamins.

Dried fruit is a good source of natural, but very concentrated, sweetness. Add dried fruits to cereals or soak them in water as a dessert, but don't eat too much of them in the dried form, because the level of sweetness is so high that it will keep alive your craving for sugar. Another good reason for not eating too much dried fruit is that much of it is treated with sulfur to keep it looking plump and glossy. Some stores now sell unsulfered dried fruit which, despite its dull, shrivelled appearance, is worth seeking out and actually tastes better. You could also look into inexpensive home devices for drying your own fruit.

29

PROTEIN

Protein is the body's building and repair nutrient. It is essential to growth. During digestion, food proteins are broken down into amino acids, chemicals which are absorbed into the body. The standard recommended requirement calls for about 12 percent, or one-eighth, of your total daily calories to be protein.

If your intake of energy foods, such as carbohydrates and fats, is insufficient, your liver will transform your body protein into glycogen, the only immediate available source of energy. Glycogen fuels the vital organs of the body: the brain, liver, heart, and so on. If your body protein must be metabolized to supply immediate energy, then its proper function with regard to growth and repair is sacrificed. This is why starvation, low-calorie, and high-protein diets, which eliminate carbohydrates, lead to the loss of lean tissue, general slowing of the metabolism, poor skin and hair, slow healing of cuts, and extreme fatigue.

Protein used to be divided into two classes: animal and vegetable. In the past, animal protein, such as meat, fish, milk, cheese, and eggs, was favored because it supplied all eight essential amino acids. Although vegetable proteins often lack one or other of these amino acids, this deficiency can be made up by eating them in the right combinations. Cereals, dried beans, nuts, rice, peas, and seeds can be combined and are all good sources of protein.

For many of us, meat conjures up the perfect picture of prime protein. In fact, this is a misconception. The usable protein content of meat is only about 25 percent, whereas soybeans can have proportionately much more. When soybeans are made into tofu (also called bean curd), its protein content is as high as 40 percent — much higher than meat.

How the protein-based food is prepared also determines the protein's effectiveness. Some meats, if overcooked, cause the digestive process to slow down. This, in turn, reduces the amount of available protein. Beans and cereals can also lose valuable protein if under- or over-cooked.

Why we need food *Everyone must eat to maintain the health of his or her body. Protein, carbohydrate and fat are the three basic ingredients of food. These supply energy and heat, and, together with vitamins and minerals, provide the raw materials for the growth and repair of cells and tissues.*

Food is chewed and swallowed.

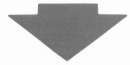

The stomach mixes the food with acid and enzymes.

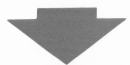

Juice from the pancreas and bile from the liver digest the large molecules in the food and break them down into smaller units.

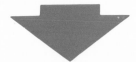

Sugars, vitamins, amino acids, fat, water and minerals are all absorbed from the small intestine and ferried to the liver by the blood.

Unabsorbed food is turned into faeces and excreted through the anus.

The kidneys filter the blood and make urine from waste chemicals and water.

The liver controls the use of all the raw materials that are absorbed by the intestine but not immediately used by the tissues. They are released into the blood or stored according to the demands of the body. Sugars are converted into glucose or glycogen, fats are broken down and stored, while surplus amino acids are turned into urea for excretion.

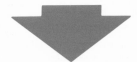

The blood carries the nutrients derived from food to all the cells of the body.

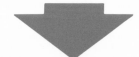

The nutrients diffuse into the cells from the blood. Once there, they are used according to their nutritional value. Sugars are the primary source of energy and heat. Amino acids are used for growth, to repair any damaged tissue or in the production of enzymes.

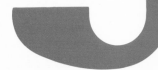

SEEDS AND SPROUTS

Since they can form such an important part of your new diet, seeds and sprouts deserve special attention. Besides being an excellent source of nourishment, they are plentiful and inexpensive compared with other protein sources. Remember that grains in their unprocessed form are also seeds. Here are some suggestions to get you started:

● Seeds that are good to eat in their natural state are: poppy, sunflower, sesame, and pumpkin. Others are usually cooked or sprouted.

● Combine sesame, sunflower, and pumpkin seeds for a delicious, crunchy breakfast topping. When combined together these three seeds make a complete protein. They provide essential fatty acids that are vital to the health; they also help to balance cholesterol levels.

● Add sunflower seeds to any cooked grain — buckwheat, for example — that already has a warm, nutty flavor, for added nourishment and texture.

● Use seeds as crunchy toppings and in salads. Remember that adding texture to foods is a good way to make them more inviting to your family.

● Make up seed, nut, and dried-fruit mixes for snacks and children's lunch boxes. It's a good idea to introduce your children to nutritionally sound foods. Encourage them to share them with their friends!

● Use poppy and sesame seeds in bread and other baking.

● All seeds and beans can be sprouted. This increases their nutritional value immensely. Add the sprouted seeds and beans to sandwiches and salads. They provide an interesting alternative to lettuce as texture-based filler. You can buy many bean sprouts and alfalfa sprouts at your supermarket. You can also sprout your own by arranging the seeds or beans on damp paper towels in a dark place. Keep the towels damp and in a few days you'll have sprouts — eat them quickly.

It's a good idea to concentrate on eating seeds and sprouts and keep your consumption of nuts low. Although peanuts, for example, are an excellent source of carbohydrates and protein, they also contain large amounts of fats and calories. Five peanuts are about 50 calories. So the next time you're munching on a snack, remember that a handful of peanuts may contain more calories than a can of sodapop or beer!

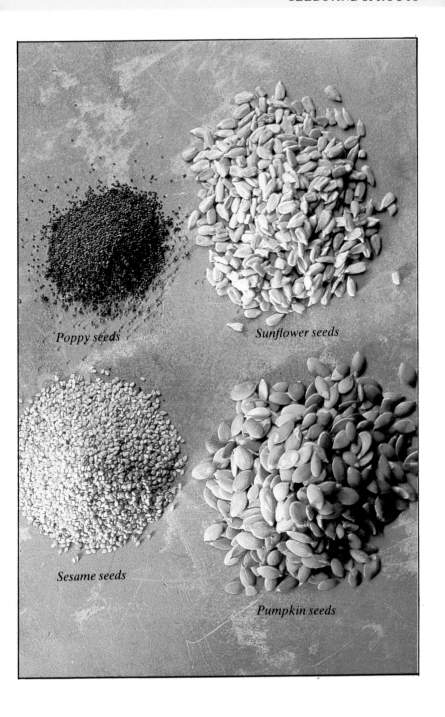

Poppy seeds

Sunflower seeds

Sesame seeds

Pumpkin seeds

WATER

The human body can survive without many nutrients for long periods, but it cannot survive for long without water. Like the planet Earth, where 75 per cent of the surface is covered by water, the human body is a walking canteen too! Most people are about 70 percent water. The brain, blood, and muscles are all one part tissue and three parts water. Water is a key ingredient as a building block of the system. In an average day, you'll need to consume almost three quarts of water. Since very few of us actually drink that much, where do we get our supply? Surprisingly, most of our water comes from the foods we eat. Fruits, vegetables, even eggs and bread contain water. Poultry, yogurt, and milk are also excellent sources of the miracle drink. The water in these foods comes as a byproduct of the body's metabolic reactions during digestion. As your body is busy turning that peanut butter and jelly sandwich into fats, protein

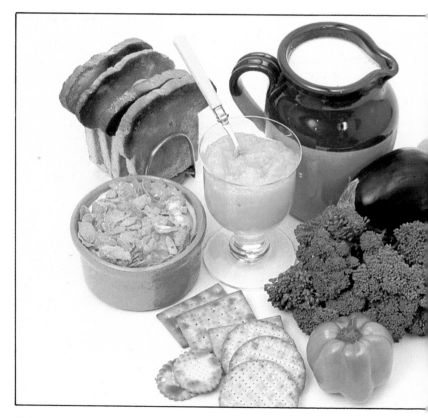

and carbohydrates, water is released and absorbed into the system.

One factor determining the amount of water you require is the amount of energy being exerted. The more you exercise and sweat, the more water has to be replaced. In hot weather, you'll have to drink more water to replenish the amount leaving your body through perspiration.

Hardly a food substance on the grocer's shelf is not made primarily of water. You should not, however, drink sugar-laced liquids to replenish water during exercise. These drinks actually take water from the tissues of the body and divert them to the stomach to help your system dilute and then drain off the sugar. So while you are trying to get water into your muscles and tissue, you are actually causing the reverse effect by further draining those already strained organs. That is why some athletes develop muscle cramps after chugging down a soft drink on the sidelines. The drink starts the internal water-draining process and soon the muscles lack water and cramps occur.

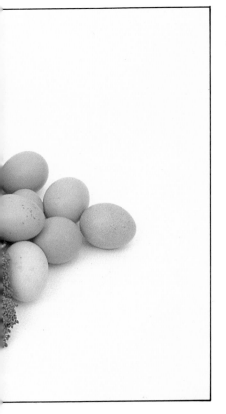

By far the greatest proportion of the water we consume comes from the foods we eat, rather than the fluids we drink.

FATS

Fats provide us with energy and help keep us warm. They are also important to our vital organs and help maintain healthy skin. However, our need for fat is minimal and a diet high in saturated fat may be a major contributory factor in the development of heart disease and some forms of cancer. The standard recommended intake of fat should be 30 percent or about one-third, of your daily calories. Of that figure, only 10 percent should be saturated fats. A diet high in vegetables, grains, nuts, seeds, and fruits provides all the fat the system needs.

Liquid and solid fats are divided into two types: saturated and unsaturated. In general, a saturated fat is thick and solid at room temperature. It comes chiefly from dairy products and meat, but another source of saturated fats is coconut and palm-kernel oil. That is why it is important to read package labels. Many so-called health foods actually contain high percentages of saturated fats in

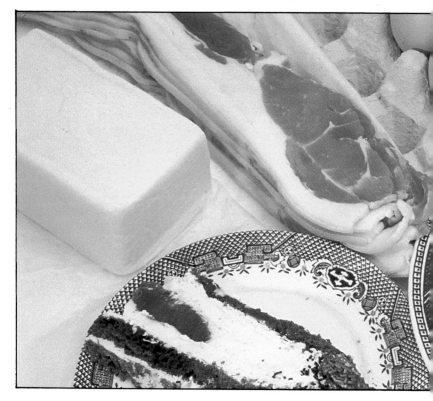

the form of these oils.

Unsaturated fats fall into two categories: mono-unsaturated fats are found in fish, poultry, some margarines, and peanut and olive oils. Polyunsaturated fats are found in certain fish and corn and safflower oils. Unsaturated fats of both kinds are thought to have a beneficial effect. They help reduce cholesterol and may therefore be useful in preventing heart disease.

Surprisingly, some of the saturated fats we consume come from very hidden sources. For example, fast foods are loaded with saturated fats. Most of it comes not from the ground beef, but from the cheese toppings, the "secret sauces," the fried potatoes, and even those milk shakes we drink to wash it all down. These food chains use saturated fats like palm and coconut oil for frying and in preparing their shakes and toppings. Lately, some of the stores have changed to healthier unsaturated fats in response to the public's growing awareness of nutrition. Next time you're at your favorite burger-on-the-run place, ask for a nutritional guide and see just what you're eating!

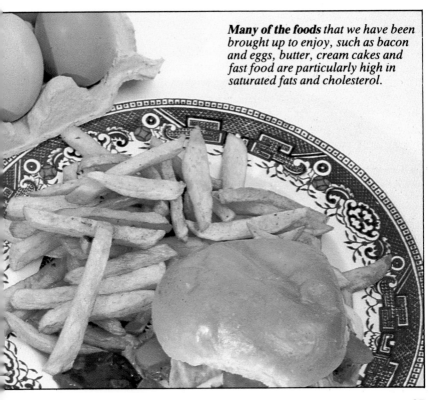

Many of the foods that we have been brought up to enjoy, such as bacon and eggs, butter, cream cakes and fast food are particularly high in saturated fats and cholesterol.

HIDDEN FAT — THE MASKED BANDIT

Nobody in her right mind would walk up to the counter at the local diner and say, "Let me have a fat sandwich with a side order of fat and a fat-shake to wash it down." Yet that is precisely what many of us do each day, merely by eating foods that contain huge amounts of hidden fat — the masked bandit. This fat hides within the safe confines of cheeses, fried foods, meat, chocolate, and dairy products.

On the average we eat about 3.5 ounces of fat each day. This amounts to around 40 percent of our total energy intake. There is substantial evidence that a more sensible amount would be half that!

Studies in a number of countries have shown that the number of people dying from heart disease and from cancers of the intestines is probably closely linked with the amount of fat and animal products that they have consumed. Although the main sources are meat, milk, butter, and cheese, some fat enters the body masked as an ingredient in processed or manufactured foods.

If you purchase manufactured foods you should read the label and check the ingredients. The label should have a breakdown of the contents, including the "fat content" of the food. If not, check the list of ingredients and look for the signs of hidden or masked fat. Things like palm oil or coconut oil are high in saturated fats. So if the front label proudly claims that it is made from 100 percent

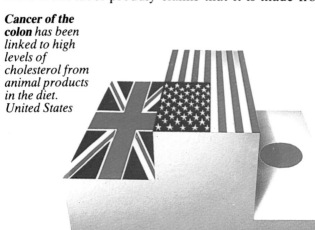

Cancer of the colon has been linked to high levels of cholesterol from animal products in the diet. United States citizens are seven times more vulnerable than those of Japan, where the consumption of animal fat is low.

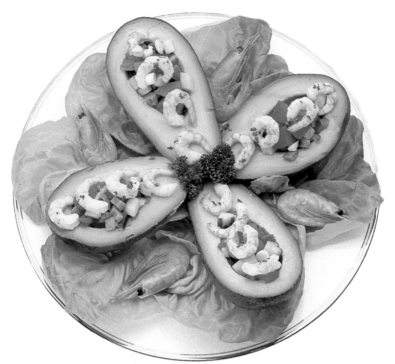

Despite their continuing popularity *as a health food, avocado pears in* *fact contain the same fat content as bacon or butter!*

vegetable oil, you'd better check to see which vegetable they're talking about!

A likely source of unwanted fat is the restaurant. Even though you go there with high ideals, hoping to eat a healthy meal, you may get held up by the masked bandit. Sure, you pass on the butter and deep-fried zucchini. But you'll destroy your chances of eating a low-fat meal as you spoon up the soup or dive into that salad with blue cheese dressing.

To keep to your goal, stay away from anything on the menu that is creamed, sautéed, fried or called "crispy." Invariably these are made with more than a little dash of the masked bandit. Of course, you'll want to eat a salad, since your new diet calls for these leafy greens to be a basic part of your food intake. But ask the waiter for an oil and vinegar dressing. In any event, request that the dressing be put on the side so that you can control the amount on your salad. And speaking of salads, the California avocado craze provides a hideout for the masked bandit. Avocados have as much fat content as bacon or butter!

CHOLESTEROL

Cholesterol is an essential element of the body found in all its tissues. It aids the formation of tissue, membranes, vitamin D, and certain nerve packages. Unfortunately, too much cholesterol may lead to clogged arteries and heart disease.

Cholesterol becomes available to the body from two sources. It is manufactured in the liver and is also consumed as part of our food intake. The main food sources are eggs, meat, cheese, butter, milk, cream, and animal fats in general. Plant foods contain no cholesterol, while the quantities in margarine may vary, depending on whether plant or animal oil is used in its manufacture. You can sharply reduce the amount of cholesterol sources, you and your liver will still produce enough to keep you healthy.

Both the type of fat in food and its quantity can affect the amount of cholesterol in the blood. The level can be lowered if less fat is eaten. Using polyunsaturated margarine or using corn, sunflower, or safflower oil for cooking can lower the cholesterol level. But beware — many margarines and vegetable oils are unsuitable because they do not contain enough polyunsaturated fats. For those people who have a tendency to be overweight, it is more sensible to eat less fat overall.

Although many people can eat foods containing a high level of cholesterol without affecting the cholesterol level in their blood, experiments have shown that others are more sensitive. People with a relative who already suffers from heart disease are advised to eat no more than two or three eggs a week, and to restrict their intake of other foods rich in cholesterol.

Interestingly, some studies have recently shown that diets high in fiber might actually reduce the cholesterol levels in the body. We know that fiber helps to reduce toxins and acids in the body by promoting bowel movements. The bile acids in the body are made primarily from cholesterol, so a high-fiber diet can help eliminate them.

We already know that meats, eggs, and butter are high in cholesterol; some products, made up from these ingredients, compound the situation. Sponge cake, that light, fluffy desert favorite, is made with many eggs — an average slice contains as much cholesterol as six ounces of beef!

An egg-rich sponge cake (opposite), *layered with cream, may look light but is packed with as much cholesterol as six ounces of meat.*

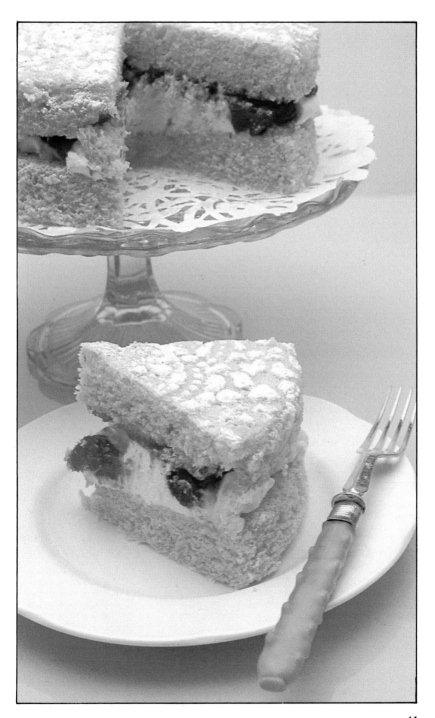

SAY HELLO TO PASTA AND POTATOES

The average person doesn't think of a potato or a plate of pasta as being complicated, but they are. They belong to a food family called complex carbohydrates — what many of us commonly call starch.

Starches are low-calorie carbohydrates that too many times are ignored by dieters. Rice, pasta, baked potatoes, and corn should be an integral part of any weight-reducing diet. They help fill you up, not out. But before you go running off to gobble down plates of lasagna and french fries, a word of caution. We recommend these starches in a fairly unadulterated form. A normal baked potato only has about 100 calories, but if you load it up with butter or sour cream, you're asking for trouble. The same holds true for pasta. An average serving of pasta has only about 200 calories, but if you add cheeses, meat sauces, and sausages, you're destroying your diet.

The trick to using these starches to help your diet is to be conservative. Instead of butter on that delicious potato, just sprinkle a little pepper on it to bring out the flavor. Surprisingly, the same condiment can be used on corn. While many of you bathe the corn with butter and salt, a little pepper brings out the vegetable's natural flavor without smothering the taste!

Recent experiments with these starches and high-carbohydrate diets show that you can actually use rice and potatoes to help you feel "full" without consuming all those calories. Try eating some whole-grain bread before sitting down for a meal. The unbuttered bread, at about 75 calories per slice, makes your stomach feel satisfied; you'll find that you'll crave less food at the table. And starches made from whole grains are packed with vitamins and nutrients. Most starches are rich in digestion-aiding fiber, besides containing protein.

So the next time you want to perk up your meal, don't forget the starch family of foods. In fact, they're so good for you that they may become regulars at your dining-room table!

Make or buy your own fresh pasta, but don't smother it with sauces if you want to lose weight.

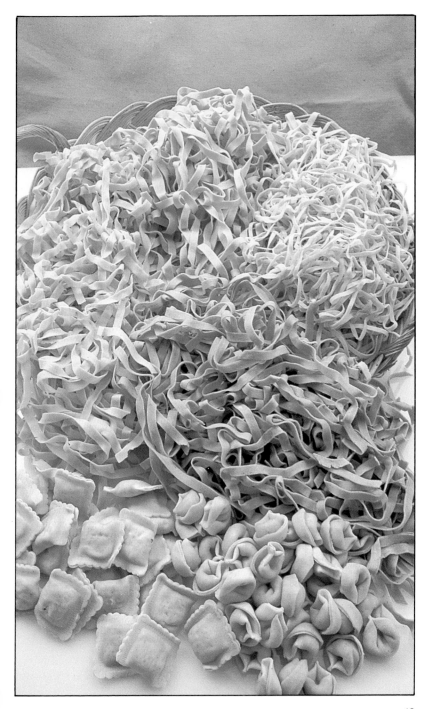

VITAMINS

Vitamins help us metabolize fats, carbohydrates, and proteins. They help maintain our tissue structure and function, keep the digestive tract working well, and help us resist infection. Certain diseases result directly from the lack of vitamins. For example, a deficiency of vitamin D, which is essential for the formation of healthy bones, can result in rickets. A low-level general vitamin deficiency can make you feel sluggish and depressed, leading perhaps to a reluctance to take exercise or binge eating to help you "get over" your depression.

There are two types of vitamins: fat-soluble, (vitamins A, D, E, and K) and water-soluble (B complex vitamins and vitamin C). Water-soluble vitamins are not stored in the body, so a daily intake is necessary. Excess water-soluble vitamins, whether from food or supplements, are simply passed out the body.

Although there are recommended minimum daily allowances for vitamins, requirements may vary from person to person, depending on their age, sex, general state of health, climate, and environment. Other factors, such as absorption, the relationship of one vitamin to another, and the intake of other nutrients, all play important roles in our body's needs.

Here are some facts and figures on vitamins:

● **VITAMIN A.** Essential for maintaining the membranes of the eyes and lungs. Helps maintain resistance to infections; necessary for the prevention of night-blindness. A good natural source of vitamin A is milk and milk products; green leafy vegetables provide the vitamin in a natural state.

● **VITAMIN B1.** Plays an important role in releasing energy from carbohydrates and maintaining the digestive system. Good sources are whole-grain cereals, fruits, nuts, and beans.

● **VITAMIN C.** Essential to the formation of healthy tissues including skin, dentine, and cartilage. Vitamin C is also important in healing wounds and fractures. Good natural sources are citrus fruits and tomatoes.

● **VITAMIN D.** Regulates absorption of calcium and phosphorus from the intestinal tract. Vitamin D is found in butter, egg yolks, liver, and fatty fish.

● **VITAMIN E.** The best-known function of vitamin E is as an antioxidant, protecting the body's polyunsaturated fats from destruction by oxygen. It also protects and preserves vitamin A. Found in lettuce, wheat germ, and sunflower oil.

VITAMINS IN THE DIET

VITAMIN A
Provitamin, carotene • Essential for maintaining such membranes as eyes and lungs • Helps maintain resistance to infections • Necessary for the formation of rhodopsin and prevention of night blindness
Good sources: butter/cheese/egg yolk/whole milk/fish liver oil/liver/green leafy vegetables/carrots/all yellow vegetables/special concentrates

VITAMIN B_1
Thiamine • Important role in releasing energy from carbohydrates • Essential for maintenance of normal digestion and appetite • Essential for normal functioning of nervous tissue.
Good sources: Widely distributed in plant and animal tissues but seldom occurs in high concentration, except in brewer's yeast. Whole grain cereals/peas, beans/peanuts/oranges/variety meats/fruits and nuts

VITAMIN B_2
Riboflavin • Important in utilization of food energy • Formation of certain enzymes and in cellular oxidation
Good sources: eggs/green vegetables/lean meat/milk/wheat germ/dried yeast/enriched foods

VITAMIN B_3
Nicotinic acid, Antipellagra vitamin • As the component of two important enzymes, it is important in glycolysis, tissue respiration, and fat synthesis • Prevents pellagra

VITAMIN B_{12}
Cyanocobalmin • Produces remission in pernicious anemia • Essential for normal development of red blood cells
Good sources: liver/kidney/dairy products

VITAMIN C
Ascorbic acid • Essential to formation of healthy tissues including skin, dentine, cartilage and bone matrix • Important in healing of wounds and fractures of bones • Prevents scurvy • Facilitates absorption of iron
Good sources: most fresh fruits and vegetables, especially citrus fruit and juices, tomato and orange

VITAMIN D
• Regulates absorption of calcium and phosphorus from the intestinal tract
Good sources: butter/egg yolk/fish liver oils/fatty fish/liver/oysters/yeast/formed in the skin by exposure to sunlight

VITAMIN E
Alpha tocopherol • The best known function of vitamin E is as an anti-oxidant — protecting the body's polyunsaturated fats from destruction by oxygen • It also protects vitamin A
Good sources: lettuce and other green leafy vegetables/wheat germ/sunflower oil/margarine/eggs/cereals/breast milk

VITAMIN B_6
Pyridozine • Metabolism of amino acids • Formation of hemoglobin.
Good sources: meat/cereal grains/wheat germ/blackstrap molasses

FOLIC ACID
Folacin • As for vitamin B_{12} essential in the formation of red blood cells • Can possibly help prevent birth defects
Good sources: variety meats/yeast/green, leafy vegetables/fruit

MINERALS

Minerals are also essential to your body. They help to maintain the water and acid–alkaline balance. They are important in the formation of tissues, blood cells, muscles, and bones. Some minerals act as a catalyst for important biochemical reactions and the production of certain hormones.

The major minerals, such as calcium, phosphorus, potassium, magnesium, and sodium, are stored in the body in amounts of five grams or more. Trace minerals, also known as micronutrients, such as zinc, sulfer, iodine, and manganese are found in the body in very minute amounts. But the distinction between major and trace minerals does not mean that the first group is more important. A daily deficiency in one of the trace minerals can be serious. Studies have shown that women tend to suffer most from deficiencies in zinc, chromium, and manganese.

Here are some food sources for important minerals:

● **PHOSPHORUS.** Essential to building and strengthening bones and teeth and maintaining cell tissues, phosphorus is found in various meats and poultry. Basics like dried beans and split peas also provide the necessary phosphorus.

● **MAGNESIUM.** Important to the development of bones and the manufacture of proteins, magnesium also serves as a catalyst in the release of energy in muscle cells. Magnesium comes from dark, leafy green vegetables and from certain nuts, such as almonds.

● **CALCIUM.** Studies show that calcium is one of the chief minerals to aid in the development and strength of bones and teeth. Also a factor in the body's ability to maintain cell tissue, calcium comes chiefly from milk and the various milk products. Certain fish, such as sardines and salmon, also provide calcium.

● **POTASSIUM.** Providing the essentials for muscle maintenance and nerve impulse transmission, potassium comes from a variety of sources, including bananas, bran, and peanut butter.

● **ZINC.** Zinc has been shown to be a major element of more than 75 of the body's enzymes. Zinc is found in liver, seafood, and eggs.

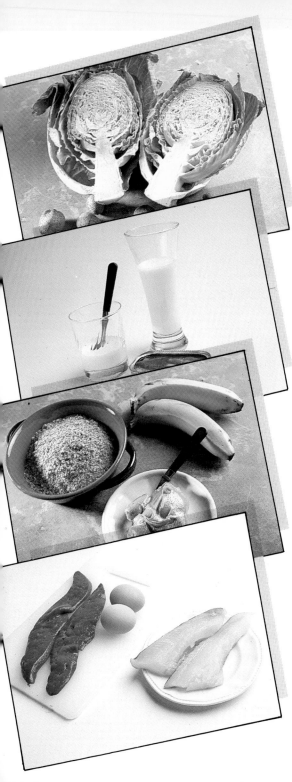

Leafy green vegetables *and some nuts, particularly almonds, are a good source of magnesium.*

The main source of calcium *in most diets is milk products. Sardines and salmon also contain valuable quantities of the mineral.*

Potassium *can be obtained from a number of sources, among which are bananas, bran and peanut butter.*

Including liver, seafood and eggs *in your diet will ensure adequate supplies of zinc.*

FIBER

Fiber, in the form of bran, cellulose, and pectin, is the indigestible part of food. It passes through the digestive tract without being absorbed. It is now generally accepted that a diet high in fiber is healthy. The fiber helps food pass quickly through the intestines and bowels, removing toxins and helping to prevent the development of such serious disorders as diverticular disease, heart disease, and certain cancers.

However, one unfortunate aspect of the attention fiber has attracted is that it is now regarded as a magic cure-all. Sales of wheat bran have shot up and people are busily sprinkling the dry flakes on soups, stews, cereals, and desserts. Unfortunately, bran consumed this way is likely to have a sudden, irritating effect on the bowels, and can cause gas.

For health and comfort you should eat a variety of fibers.

Of all the conclusions that researchers have drawn about how we can look after our figure and health by changing our eating habits, the realization of the importance of fiber — found in such foods as pulses and vegetable produce — is perhaps the most significant. Diverticular disease, heart disease and certain cancers have all been linked to a lack of fiber in the diet. Moreover, fiber not only fills us up, reducing appetite, but also ensures that energy from food is absorbed more slowly — staving off hunger pangs.

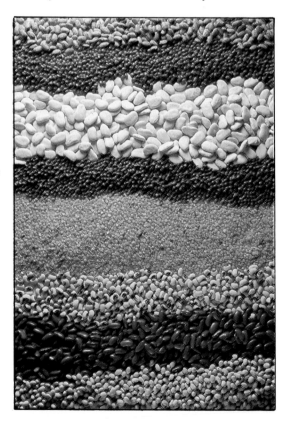

Focusing on fiber as something separate from the rest of the food we eat is not very helpful. A healthy diet should consist of a range of good food in as whole a state as possible. Concentrate on eating whole grains, fruits and a wide range of vegetables to ensure the best possible diet, and you'll get lots of fiber naturally.

Increasing the fiber content in your food helps you slim in two ways. Firstly, high-fiber foods generally contain fewer calories but more bulk than the same amount of low-fiber foods; they also need more chewing. This helps you feel fuller and so reduces your appetite. Secondly high-fiber food reduces the energy absorbed from food, while also ensuring that the energy that is absorbed gets absorbed more slowly.

Since the cell walls of virtually all plants contain fiber, vegetables and fruits are an excellent source of dietary fiber. However, the best source is still whole grain products like bran, cereals, and even whole meal pasta. For example, one cup of bran flakes cereal contains 12 times more fiber than one cup of raw cauliflower.

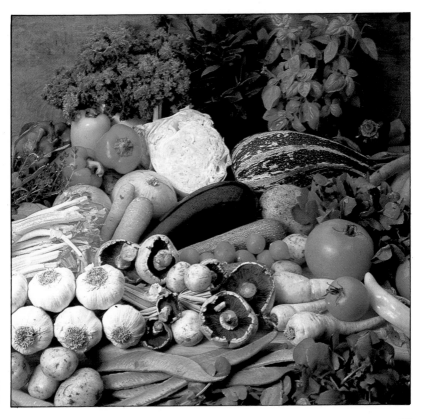

S<u>ALT</u>

Your body requires very little salt to maintain its functioning chemistry. Despite this fact, most people eat considerable amounts of salt, both in cooking and at the table. And if you read the label on processed food (a very good habit to get into), you'll see that many manufacturers add salt to their foods. Sometimes it is used as a preservative, but more often it is added to enhance the taste. Salt

Experiment with garlic and lemon juice to season food, instead of using salt.

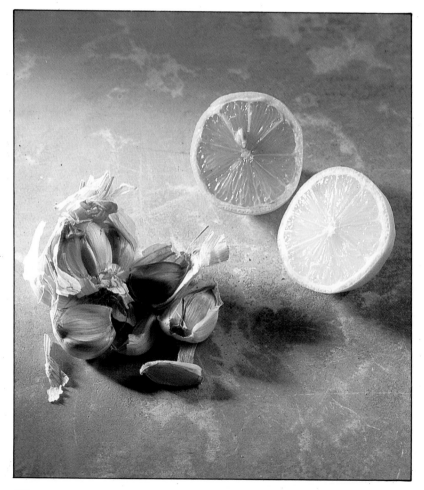

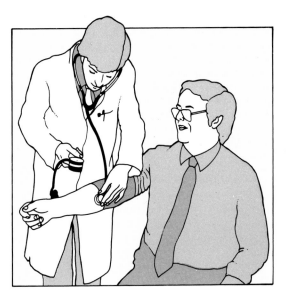

Most doctors now regularly screen their older patients for hypertension (high blood pressure), a condition which predisposes a person to strokes and heart disease. A reduction in salt intake is usually advised if the blood pressure is found to be raised.

is present in bread, butter, and margarine. Monosodium glutamate, another type of salt, is added to virtually all "convenience foods" and is a staple in most Chinese diets. Unprocessed food, however, contains very little salt.

Hypertension, or high blood pressure, can be a symptom of a number of medical conditions, or a disease itself. In many people with a family history of hypertension, there seems to be a relationship between a high level of salt in the diet and high blood pressure. A proportion of people seem to be particularly sensitive to this.

Since hypertension markedly increases the probability of a stroke and is a major risk factor in heart disease, most doctors now screen their patients for the problem. Part of the treatment for those with high blood pressure is a reduction in the intake of salt. Table salt should not be used, and it should be omitted entirely in cooking. It's surprising how quickly you can get used to far less salt in your diet. In fact, once you put away your salt shaker you may find that food in restaurants, for example, suddenly tastes salty.

Instead of salt, try lemon juice, garlic, and spices to season your food.

If you intend to cut back on salt, read the labels on bottles and cans. Processed soups, long thought to be delicious and nutritious, often contain vast amounts of salt. Some soup manufacturers have introduced low-sodium products. Look for them and ladle them up! Another way to help keep your salt intake down is stop eating pickles, ketchup, and other condiments that frequently have a high salt content.

SUGAR — EMPTY CALORIES

Sugar, whether white or brown, is a major ingredient of cookies, cakes, biscuits, ice cream, soft drinks and many other foods. But sugar is an "empty calorie" food, providing energy but no other nutrients. Sugar also promotes tooth decay. Sugar has become less popular as people realize how harmful it can be.

Eating a lot of sugar in concentrated form — an ice-cream cone, for example — means that too much sugar enters the bloodstream too quickly; your blood sugar level shoots up. The pancreas, which deals with the disposition of glucose in the body, is alerted; it panics and secretes large quantities of insulin to deal with the overload. The sugar is then disposed of rapidly. Some goes into the liver as glycogen, but a great deal more is converted into the low-density lipoproteins that have been implicated in heart disease; from there they become body fat.

Because of the panic reaction of the pancreas, this disposal job is too efficient. Very soon, the blood sugar level plummets to below the level needed for well-being. So the end result is that a few hours later after your sugary snack, you're feeling hungry again!

If you respond to the hunger by eating more sugary food, the process is once more set in motion. This exhausts the body's internal alarm system — the hormone adrenaline — which sounds the alarm whenever the body is dangerously short of glucose. Eating properly will help keep your blood sugar levels stable.

In the short-term, sugary treats disrupt the body's metabolism. In the long-term, excessive sugar intake may lead to tooth decay, obesity and heart disease.

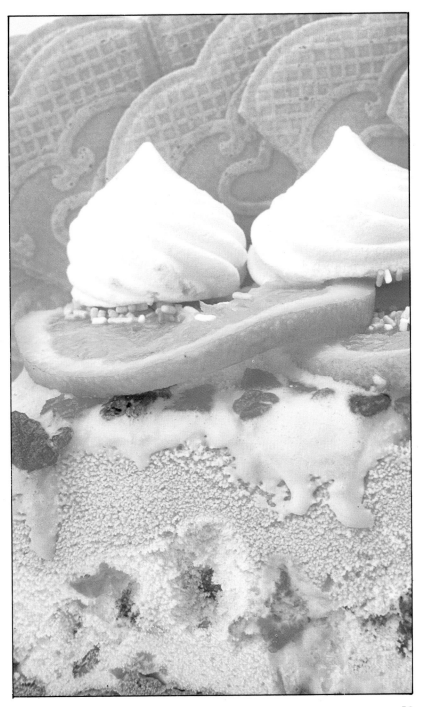

VARIETY IN YOUR DIET

A sensible diet should contain all the most important sources of each nutrient. Bread, milk, cheese, and meat contain the most protein, although they are high in fat. Oranges are high in vitamin C and carrots have the most vitamin A. Dairy fats supply vitamin A, so it is important that dark, green vegetables or carrots are eaten regularly to make up for the reduced intake of cheese, butter, eggs and cream. Similarly, whole-grain cereals, nuts, and seeds should be eaten to make up for the reduced amounts of meat protein, as well as for their fiber content.

The wider the variety of your diet, the easier it'll be to maintain it until you become a thinner, healthier person. Nobody wants to spend the rest of her life on a diet! Be creative. Once you have learned which items provide the best nourishment in each food group, experiment to come up with some new favorite recipes to keep your family happy and alive.

Speaking of food groups, remember that if one nutrient group is

A sensible diet

	Energy (kJs)	Protein (g)	Fat (g)
Breakfast			
Wheatflakes 35gm (1.4oz)	507	4.0	1.2
Sugar 5gm (0.2oz)	63		
5 slices wholemeal bread	1892	18.4	5.7
Thinly spread butter, for 5 slices			145
Marmalade 20gm (0.8oz)	218		
Milk, for cereal and drinks during the day. 450g (0.75 pint)	1214	14.8	17.1
Lunch			
1 small slice of chicken 30gm (1.2oz)	176	7.4	1.6
1 small slice of cheese 30gm (1.2oz)	498	7.8	10.0
Lettuce, tomato 100gm (4oz)	59	0.9	
Small piece fruit cake 40gm (1.6oz)	599	2.0	5.2
Fresh orange 120gm (4.8oz)	176	1.0	
Dinner			
Lentil soup, no fat, 200gm (8oz)	389	7.1	0.3
2 thin pork escalopes, 50gm (2oz)	465	16.1	5.3
Mushroom sauce 100gm (4oz)	218	1.1	3.8
Large jacket potato, 250gm (10oz)	854	3.5	0.2
Peas (2oz)	88	2.5	0.2
Carrots 100gm (4oz)	79	0.6	
Stewed apple 150gm (6oz)	377	0.4	
Natural yoghurt 100gm (4oz)	218	5.0	1.0
Nut topping 10gm (0.4oz)	218	1.1	5.2
Total (rounded up)	8914	94	73

supplying more than 25 percent of your diet, then you're probably not eating properly. You should only be eating a certain number of calories each day, so spread them around! If you're eating too many carbohydrates, cut down on the pasta. By keeping your meals well-planned, your family won't suffer from an overload of one specific group, which could lead them to snack on the side or eat away from home.

Remember that processed, manufactured food tends to have fewer nutrients than fresh, raw food. If you are trying to save money by buying canned goods, you may have to supply a vitamin supplement to your family to make up for the deficiency. In response to the new, health-conscious society, more and more supermarkets are stocking their shelves with lots of fresh produce. Do some comparative shopping and you'll find that you may save even more money by buying fresh foods and preparing them yourself. The only way to keep food additives out and to know for sure what goes into your family's stomachs is to cook from scratch. It might take a little time, but the results are healthy, tasty, vitamin-sufficient meals!

Starch (g)	Sugar (g)	Fiber (g)	Cholesterol (mg)	Calcium (mg)	Magnesium (mg)	Iron (mg)	Zinc (mg)	Vitamin B1 (mg)	Vitamin B2 (mg)	Vitamin C (mg)	Vitamin A (mg)
23.3	2.1	4.4		11	42	2.6	0.7	0.09	0.02		
	5.0										
33.3	4.4	17.8		48	195	5.2	4.2	0.55	0.13		
0.1	16.4		46	3							166
	14.4	0.1		7		0.1				2	2
	63	540	54	0.2	1.6	0.18	0.86	7	173		
			22	3	7	0.2	0.5	0.02	0.06		
			21	240	75	0.1	1.2	0.01	0.15		103
	2.8	1.5		13	11	0.4	0.2	0.06	0.04	20	
6.0	17.2	1.2	16	24	10	0.6	0.2	0.04	0.02		
	10.2	1.8		49	16	0.4	0.2	0.08	0.02	46	7
15.2	0.7	3.5		12	23	2.3	0.9	0.15	0.06		3
			55	4	15	0.6	1.7	0.44	0.13		
0.8	3.1			30	4	0.3	0.3		0.05		
51.0	1.5	6.0		6	37	0.7	0.5	0.25	0.10	15	
0.5	1.7	2.5		15	11	0.7	0.3	0.12	0.03	7	50
0.1	4.2	3.1		37	6	0.4	0.3	0.05	0.04	4	2000
	23.4	2.4		21	30	0.3	0.1	0.03	0.03	16	4
	6.2		7	180	17	0.1	0.6	0.05	0.26		6
0.2	0.3	0.5		6	13	0.2	0.3	0.03	0.01		
190	114	45	230	1249	566	15	14	2	2	117	2624

THE DANGERS OF CRASH DIETING

Your body is a fine-tuned machine that needs fuel to keep it going. The fuel, in the form of nutrients, is usually supplied by the food you eat, which must first of all be digested and broken down into its component parts. A peanut butter and jelly sandwich soon becomes simple fats, proteins, and carbohydrates. These nutrients are either stored for later use or sent packing through the intestines for removal.

What makes the human body unique is its ability to adapt to certain short-term shortages of certain nutrients. The body, for example, stores energy as fat. If there is a demand for energy and the fuel hasn't been supplied by food, the body will tap into its storage and break down the fat.

Take, for example, what happens when you go on a semi-starvation or crash diet to shed a few pounds. When you stop eating, the body doesn't immediately start to burn up fat for energy. The first compounds that get absorbed are water and your blood sugar, known as glucose, which comes from glycogen.

Glycogen is the body's immediate available source of energy. It is stored in the muscles and other vital organs. It is essential to the body, providing the instant energy required for all your actions, from running a mile to lifting a coffee mug.

If you crash diet, you may lose some weight, but the body must replace glycogen quickly once it is used, particularly after intense effort, illness, or a crash diet and the benefit is likely to last only a short time because of the body's natural compensating reactions. Hence the cravings, thirst, and disturbed eating habits, such as the ravenous hunger and gorging, which often take place after a starvation diet. The body is protecting itself by responding to the altered blood sugar levels; when they fall too low the appestat, the hunger control center in the brain, is triggered and you feel hungry.

When you stop dieting, your body will first replace the glycogen and water as quickly as possible; then it will replenish its "food stores." If you are an inactive person, your body has no great need for a lot of lean tissue, since muscles burn more calories than fat and therefore need more feeding. So the body will replace the lost weight with fat rather than lean tissue. Your crash diet has actually made you heavier.

Any sensible diet must take into account the body's adaptability. You must train your system to expect and cope with a smaller quantity of food.

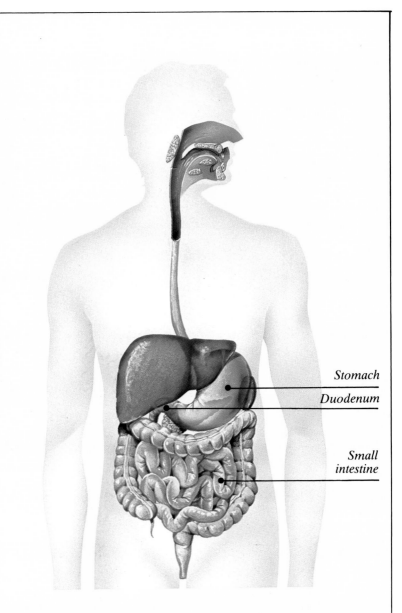

Stomach

Duodenum

Small
intestine

Food is broken down into its component parts *at a number of different stages during digestion. A crash diet alters the normal absorption of nutrients, with the eventual result that when eating returns to normal the lost weight is quickly replaced by fat rather than lean tissue.*

KEEP A CALORIE COUNT

Since part of our approach to losing weight and maintaining your weight loss is based on calorie intake, start keeping a record of what you eat. Beginners often assume that they can remember what they had during the day. But they may forget one or two items, like that extra bowl of granola for breakfast, and soon, because they're not losing weight, they go back to their old, unhealthy eating habits.

The best way to keep track of what you eat, at least until your system is accustomed to the new diet, is to record everything you eat right after it's consumed. We don't mean that you sit at the table writing, "one tablespoon of oatmeal" followed by "another tablespoon of oatmeal." Instead, after every meal, write down what you ate, including any seasonings or condiments.

What this record will do for you is give you a constant incentive to keep losing weight. You'll find that creativity will come into play as you get tired of writing down the same low-calorie foods every day. Soon, you'll naturally be selecting the proper foods in the proper amounts and you won't need to keep the record.

In the beginning, make it a habit of tallying the day's calorie intake before going to bed (many inexpensive books giving calorie counts for common foods are easily available). Write the total on the bottom on the page and next to it your weight. Then, as the weeks go by, you can easily flip through the book and see how your weight has dropped, giving you even more incentive to continue!

Another advantage of keeping this calorie count is that you'll soon begin to see the results of a few bad eating habits. For example, maybe at work you traditionally have a pastry with your morning coffee. If you've adopted our diet plan and already had your breakfast at home, you can easily do without the pastry. If you feel that you deserve a reward for arriving at work, treat yourself to a piece of fruit. If that proves too unsettling, then cut out the strawberry-cheese Danish and instead nibble on an unbuttered, whole-wheat roll. Most people don't even remember (or should that be they try to forget!) eating these little snacks during the day. But if you enter them in your calorie record, you won't be able to forget and soon you won't even want them!

THE RULES OF HEALTHY EATING

Increasing the fiber content in your food helps you slim in two ways. Firstly, high-fiber food generally contains fewer calories, but more bulk, than the same amount of low-fiber food. Secondly, high-fiber food reduces the energy absorbed from food.

Food	Percentage
Wheatbran	44.0
Haricot beans (uncooked)	25.4
Butterbeans (uncooked)	21.6
Puffed wheat	15.4
Almonds	14.3
Coconut (fresh)	13.6
Crispbread	11.7
Cornflakes	11.0
Wholemeal flour	9.6
Peanuts	8.1
Peas (uncooked frozen)	7.8
Brown flour (85%)	7.5
Muesli	7.4
Raisins (dried)	6.8
Spinach	6.3
Sweetcorn (canned)	5.7
Brown rice	5.5
Brown bread	5.1
Spring greens (boiled)	3.8
Lentils (boiled)	3.7
Bananas	3.4
Carrots (boiled)	3.1
White flour	3.0
Cabbage (boiled)	2.5
Apples (peeled)	2.0
Oranges	2.0
Tomatoes (fresh)	1.5
Lettuce	1.5
Potatoes (boiled)	1.0
White rice (boiled)	0.8
Porridge (cooked)	0.8

Which foods contain fiber? The chart (*above*) shows the percentage fiber content of some popular foods.

SPECIAL INGREDIENTS

Until quite recently, salads tended to consist of a tasteless concoction of lettuce, tomato and cucumber and were served only on hot summer days. Now, because they spell "health", salads are at the peak of their popularity — and they are eaten all through the year. They are many and varied and can include more or less any ingredient. All that is required is a little imagination and willingness to experiment. The most popular salads such as salade nicoise from France (with lettuce, tuna, olives, and hard-cooked eggs), Greek Salad (with feta cheese, tomatoes, onions and olives) and Waldorf Salad (with apples, celery, walnuts and dates), always have a pleasing balance of color, flavor and texture so that they appeal both to the eye and to the palate.

Here are some less obvious ingredients that can be used successfully in salads. Nuts, for instance, are an often-neglected food and are versatile enough to be used in many types of salad.

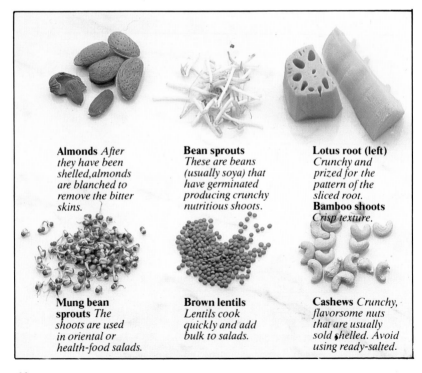

Almonds *After they have been shelled, almonds are blanched to remove the bitter skins.*

Bean sprouts *These are beans (usually soya) that have germinated producing crunchy nutritious shoots.*

Lotus root (left) *Crunchy and prized for the pattern of the sliced root.*
Bamboo shoots *Crisp texture.*

Mung bean sprouts *The shoots are used in oriental or health-food salads.*

Brown lentils *Lentils cook quickly and add bulk to salads.*

Cashews *Crunchy, flavorsome nuts that are usually sold shelled. Avoid using ready-salted.*

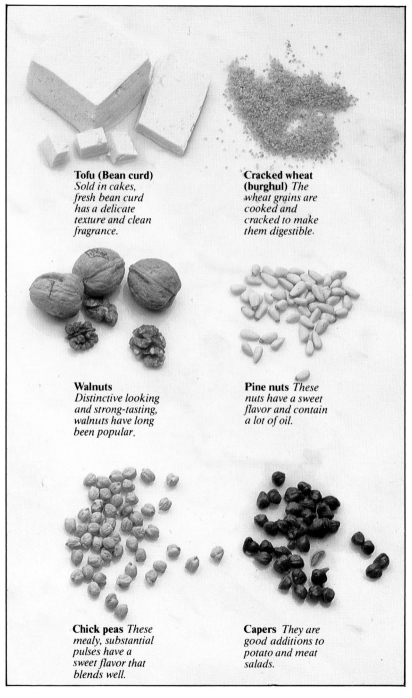

Tofu (Bean curd)
Sold in cakes, fresh bean curd has a delicate texture and clean fragrance.

Cracked wheat (burghul) *The wheat grains are cooked and cracked to make them digestible.*

Walnuts
Distinctive looking and strong-tasting, walnuts have long been popular.

Pine nuts *These nuts have a sweet flavor and contain a lot of oil.*

Chick peas *These mealy, substantial pulses have a sweet flavor that blends well.*

Capers *They are good additions to potato and meat salads.*

CHANGING YOUR EATING STYLE

Very few of us like to make public announcements about being on a diet. You're at a dinner party and while most people are gorging themselves on lasagna and apple pie à la mode, you sit quietly at the table, almost embarrassed, as you pick at your salad with low-calorie dressing and an apple without the à la mode. So what can you do? What you can do is begin to change your way of thinking about food!

Since you've incorporated our plan of losing weight by reducing your daily calorie intake, while still eating from the major food groups, your diet is going to work! Unlike some of your friends, who are always going on one gimmick diet after another, you are determined to lose the weight and not to let it creep back on again. You have to begin to think differently about food and your eating habits.

Just as your car's fuel tank can only hold so much gasoline, the

---

GIMMICK DIETS

You got on the scale this morning, you're a few pounds over-weight, and it's time to start a sensible diet. Now what do you do? Unfortunately, if you're like most people, you begin one of the many common gimmick or fad diets. One hint to the success rates of these diets is their overabundance. There are hundreds of these diets on the market, not because of their remarkable success, but because they rarely work in the long run. Sure, you may lose a few pounds initially, but soon your body may weaken from an overload of the gimmick's food — grapefruit, for example — and you'll be back to your old eating habits. The only sensible way to diet is to reduce your calorie intake gradually while eating foods selected from all the major food groups.

Since no two individuals have the same dietary needs or tastes in foods, try making up your own low-calorie eating schedule. Make a list of those foods you like to eat. Then erase the ones that are high in calories or have large pecentages of unhealthy ingredients like fats and cholesterol. Look for calorie-saving steps that can be introduced to keep your meals under control. For example, try substituting low-fat yogurt in those recipes that call for sour cream. If you crave potatoes, bake them — don't fry them. If you haven't done so already, begin to introduce fresh

---

human body needs only so much food. The difference is that if you try to put extra gasoline in your car it spills on the ground, but if you "tank up" on extra food, it just spills onto your waist, buttocks, thighs, and chin! Learn to be a nutritional economist. Eat only what your body needs, and even then select the "low-octane" or low-calorie foods.

Since our eating habits start to develop during infancy, it'll be difficult at first to make the needed changes. You might need incentives to break your bad eating routines. Try cutting out pictures of your favorite athletes and taping them to your refrigerator. Get into the habit of weighing yourself every morning. Start looking for the new outfit you're going to buy as a reward once you shed those extra pounds.

You're not just losing weight . . . you're starting to eat healthier, more nutritious meals. Once you get into your new diet, the rest comes easy. You'll feel more alive, more energetic. Don't think of yourself as being on a diet . . . you're changing your eating style and your life!

fruits and vegetables into your family's menu. Since your goal is slowly to reduce the amount of calories you consume each day, consult a calorie chart, or better yet, keep one posted in the kitchen.

By eating from the wide range of foods available in the basic food groups, you won't be depriving your body of necessary vitamins and nutrients, as you would by going on one of those gimmick diets. The human body is like the engine of your car. Your car's engine needs water, oil, antifreeze, and gasoline to run properly. Likewise, your body needs a combination of protein, carbohydrates, water, and fats.

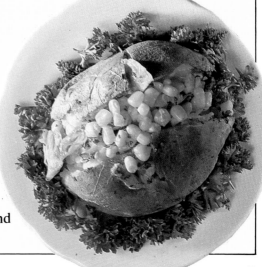

LOOK FOR YOUR BINGE TRIGGER

One way to begin to cut down your calorie intake is to recognize that certain events trigger your food binges. It's Saturday afternoon and your favorite football team is playing on national television. You run down to your local tavern, promising yourself on the way to drink club soda or maybe some low-calorie beer. Arriving at this mecca of America, you're soon cheering with the rest of the crowd. As your team scores the first touchdown, you celebrate by grabbing a fistful of salted pretzels and jamming them in your mouth. Still caught up in the frenzy, you order a "real" beer to wash it down. Soon your calorie intake is mounting as rapidly as the score. By the time the opposing team kicks the winning field goal with only seconds remaining in the game, you feel bloated and depressed. Not only has your team blown another contest, but you're also headed for the loser's locker room. Sitting at home, you realize that to make up for the gorged calories, you'd have to give up eating for a week. What happened?

What happened was that you gave in to one of your eating binge triggers. It can happen to any of us. Certain events in life can trigger eating frenzy. Some people can't resist eating popcorn and candy at the movies. Others simply must have a few snacks during car trips. It happens to all of us, but if you learn to recognize the triggering signals, you can prevent the diet-busting binges.

Make a list of all the times, besides during meals, when you have the urge to eat. For the first few days of your new eating regimen, you'll be surprised how often these urges occur.

Once you have realized when these triggering signs occur, you can take steps to avoid them. Becoming aware of the signs is the first step. If you habitually munch pretzels and peanuts at your local tavern, try placing yourself away from that bowl of calories. If that doesn't work, some people have sucess chewing on a toothpick. Sometimes eating binge food is just a nervous habit and the toothpick, simulating the chewing motion, suppresses the urge to eat.

If there are times when you simply must have something to eat, try to select foods that are nutritious and low-calorie. Take along some fruit to the movies and eat that instead of the salted, buttered popcorn. Instead of slurping down soda in the darkened theater, bring a container of orange juice. Then, as you slip down in your seat avoiding another attack by The Beast From The Deep, you can soothe your nerves with a healthy gulp of vitamin C!

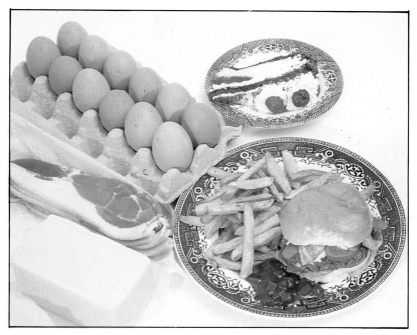

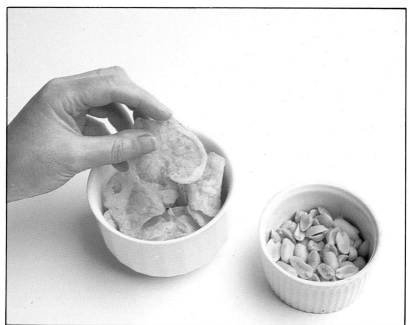

Certain occasions suggest certain foods —bacon and eggs for breakfast or peanuts with a drink — but these are often not the healthiest options.

65

THE IMPORTANCE OF BREAKFAST

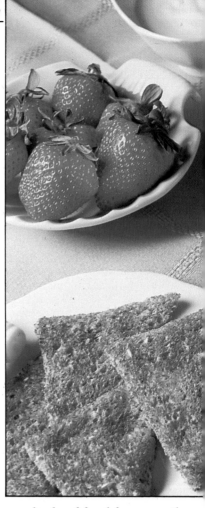

When you were a young child, your mother probably told you to "eat your breakfast, it's the most important meal of the day." That was pretty hard to believe, considering your breakfast might well have been a bowl of soggy, star-shaped marshmallows floating in a mixture of milk and sugar-coated crunchy things. But even that relatively unhealthy meal kept you going until lunch.

Breakfast is important because it can set the mood for the entire day. Without breakfast, your system may feel sluggish, your thinking dull. Remember, food is the fuel your body needs to function properly. No fuel and, like a car running out of gas, you begin to slow down.

You've been sleeping for eight hours before the day begins. Now it's time to get some food under your belt. If you don't eat anything substantial until lunch, then you've deprived your body of food for more than half a day. It's unhealthy to confine your eating to only a few hours a day. The digestive system continues to function even without fresh supplies of food, causing our stomach acids to be churned up. Tests have shown that it is better to eat several small meals spread out during the day than two large meals spaced only hours apart.

Now that you're convinced that eating a healthy breakfast is a good idea, what can you eat? Luckily, your new diet plan allows you a wide range of foods. Be creative. It is not written in stone that breakfast must consist of juice, cereal, and a piece of toast. Since you're now aware of the benefits from each food group, use

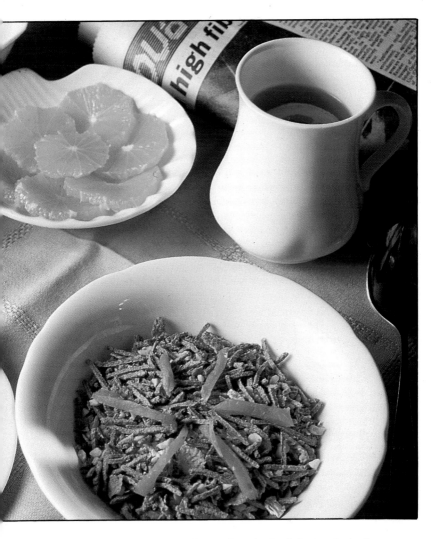

Breakfast *is just as important as the other meals of the day and what better way to start than with your* *favorite fresh fruit, wholewheat toast, mixed bran cereal and yogurt.*

your imagination to make breakfast a treat for your family. Of course, you should always supply some juice at breakfast. Keep in mind that it doesn't have to be orange juice.

If your family is growing tired of the standard breads and cereals, give them their carbohydrate fix by providing a cold pasta salad for breakfast. Remember, eating is an acquired habit and there isn't a rule that says a food can be served only for lunch or dinner!

DON'T BE A DIETING YO-YO

You can always tell people who are constantly on diets — they're the ones with two sets of clothes. When they've lost weight and are feeling good about themselves, they wear tight-fitting pants and sweaters. Then they seem to disappear from the scene for a few weeks, only to reappear wearing billowing shirts and loose-fitting skirts. Ask them about that great-looking pants suit and they'll mumble something about it "being at the cleaners." Or at least that's what you think they mumbled, since it was hard to hear what they said through their mouthful of chocolate. You have befriended a classic dieting yo-yo.

For these people, alternating diets and binges are a way of life. Their bodies are constantly fluctuating between and ideal weight and some form of obesity. Their weight goes up and down like a child's yo-yo. As their weight changes so does their personality, alternating between being outgoing and reclusive.

Besides these personality changes, scientific studies show that such fluctuations of weight can lead to serious medical problems. Repeatedly losing and gaining weight may increase the risk of heart disease. What happens is that your heart adjusts to supplying blood to a body that's one size, only to be strained to pump some more as weight is gained. A person whose weight fluctuates a lot therefore risks putting an unnecessary strain on the heart. In addition, since most of this weight gain is by fat accumulation, and fat comes primarily from unhealthy sources of food, this yo-yo person is probably consuming foods high in saturated fats and cholesterol. These items, as we now know, can lead to additional heart and circulation problems.

The only way to stop being a dieting yo-yo is to take off the additional weight sensibly and then go on a maintenance program. A maintenance program is designed to let you eat a little more food than a diet without putting on the pounds. Since we know that reduced calories leads to weight loss, it's only natural that there must be some level where you neither gain nor lose. It's a trial-and-error process, since all of us metabolize food at different rates. For example, if you've been losing weight by eating 2,000 calories a day, and you've reached your ideal weight, try increasing your diet to 2,500 calories. After a few days of adjustment, weigh yourself. If you've put on a few pounds, then cut back to 2,250 calories and see what happens. Eventually, you'll find the right amount of calories for you to maintain your weight and prevent the yo-yo syndrome.

HOW YOUR DIET CAN CAUSE A HEART ATTACK

A diet rich in saturated fats allows these to build up in your artery walls. This narrows them, slows down the blood flow, and increases the risk of blood clots forming and blocking an artery. If such a blockage occurs in one of the arteries of the heart, a heart attack is the usual result.

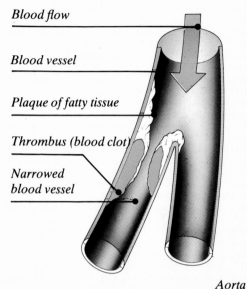

Blood flow

Blood vessel

Plaque of fatty tissue

Thrombus (blood clot)

Narrowed blood vessel

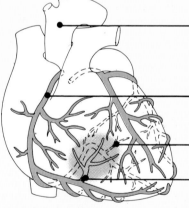

Aorta

Coronary artery

Area of muscle deprived of blood

Thrombus causing obstruction

Dieting yo-yos run a special risk of causing heart damage, so watch out for the symptoms of such diet-busting — periodic chocolate binges are a typical sign!

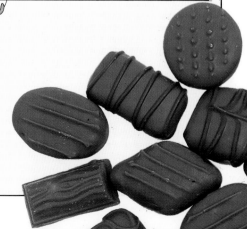

YOU CAN BE TOO THIN

Being overweight is not advisable, but neither is dropping below your ideal weight. Going overboard when trying to lose weight can cause health problems.

Body shape has always been a preoccupation, and the current obsession is with being thin — sometimes too thin. Unfortunately, some people carry dieting to the extreme and develop anorexia nervosa and bulimia, both serious eating disorders. Persons with these problems usually think they look fat, even though they may be thin, and have an abnormal fear of being fat. Common symptoms of persons suffering from anorexia and/or bulimia are bizarre food habits, refusal to eat, bingeing or gorging followed by vomiting, abuse of laxatives and diuretics, and an almost compulsive urge to exercise. Such practices can result in starvation and other chronic health problems.

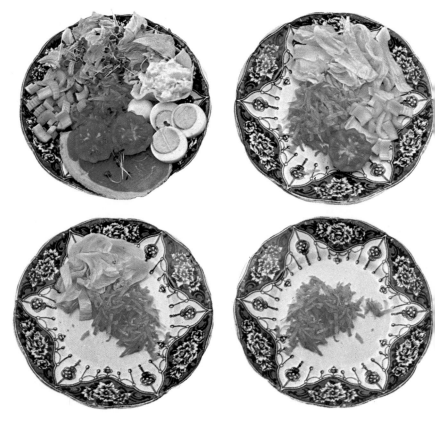

Those who suffer from anorexia will, in the first stages of the illness, feel that they are overweight even if they are aware that they are lighter than other people. They will exclude all weight-increasing foods from their diet and, even when they become so thin that the hands and feet are always cold and bones protruding, they will not want to eat more.

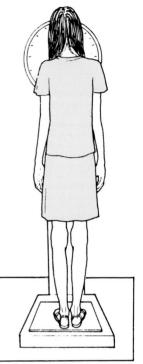

For most of us, who aren't anorexic or bulimic, the problem results more from a lack of awareness of what weight is good for our specific body types. As we begin our diet, we need to look at why we want to be thin, how thin we want to become, what methods we use to achieve this, and whether we are using our energies to pursue an illusion. Frankly, some of us may function better with a few extra pounds. Remember we all have different requirements.

Take a good look at yourself. Are you really overweight, or do you just need exercise to tighten up a little? If you are unsure, go on a diet and begin to do light exercises. Soon you should begin to see a new you!

The fact is that being underweight, or even carrying too little body fat, can be as unhealthy as being overweight or obese. For women, having too little body fat can affect their periods, their chances of becoming pregnant, and their chances of miscarrying. Statistics show that for both men and women, being too thin may mean less resistance to disease and infection, fewer resources when fighting illness, deficient nutritional intake, and even a risk of heart disease.

EARLY PREGNANCY AND NUTRITION

Three to six months before you plan to conceive you should begin thinking seriously about your diet, especially if you do not usually pay attention to eating regular, balanced meals. The future health of your baby can largely depend on giving your own body good nourishment from a time well before the fertilization of the egg. If you do not, you may actually reduce your chances of conceiving, because the hypothalamus gland in the brain responds to vitamin deficiency by suppressing the release of the hormones responsible for fertility!

Vitamin A, vitamin B6, folic acid, and the minerals zinc and magnesium are particularly important. Folic acid, a B vitamin, is essential to the manufacture of DNA and RNA, the genetic material of the cell. Zinc, found in leafy green vegetables and whole-wheat bread, is the mineral most often mentioned not only in connection with pregnancy but also for women generally, particularly since it has now been shown that a large proportion of the population is deficient in it.

Zinc plays a part in many body processes, among them the absorption of minerals and other vitamins, notably folic acid. A deficiency of it in pregnant women has been linked with the incidence of spina bifida in the baby. The official recommendation is that pregnant women need 20 milligrams of zinc daily, but much higher levels, such as 100 milligrams daily, can have a curative effect on problems such as skin disorders and water retention. Zinc is found in whole grains and meat. Zinc and calcium are also thought to provide us with some protection.

Once the baby is born, you should begin the process of proper feeding. Healthy eating habits are formed in babyhood. The way you feed your baby is therefore crucial, not only in helping it to grow healthy and strong, but in the foundation you lay down for the food choices she or he will make as an adolescent and adult. Choose baby foods that are salt- and sugar-free. Do not add sugar and salt to any food you prepare for the baby yourself, even if the food seems to be very bland. Many poor eating habits are acquired during infancy!

Vegetables such as cabbages (opposite) are an excellent source of zinc.

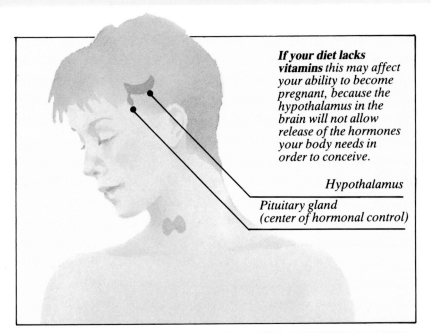

If your diet lacks vitamins this may affect your ability to become pregnant, because the hypothalamus in the brain will not allow release of the hormones your body needs in order to conceive.

Hypothalamus

Pituitary gland
(center of hormonal control)

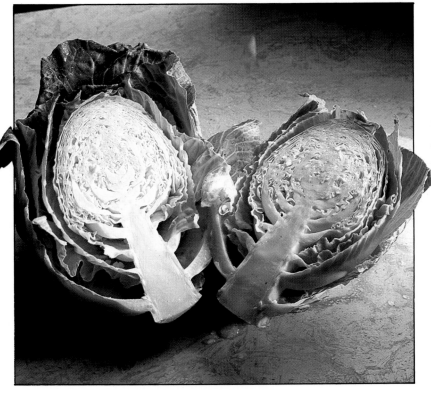

NUTRITION AND THE OLDER WOMAN

Many women over 50 face special problems. This is a time when their children have left home and many of them lose their husbands. Over a third of all women over 75 live alone. When you are no longer cooking for loved ones, there is a tendency to lose interest in food, to become careless about eating properly, and to resort to more convenience and snack foods.

When nutritional eating takes a back seat, deficiencies can develop. A shortage of vitamin C in the diet is common among older people; scurvy can even occur. To ensure that you are getting enough vitamin C, and especially if you are in this age group, eat a fresh salad every day and plenty of fruit.

It has been shown lately that zinc is vitally important to older people. Our bones become increasingly brittle as we age due to lowered calcium absorption; zinc assists calcium metabolism and helps keep bones strong. Calcium is also depleted from the body through lack of exercise. Therefore exercise is essential to maintain healthy muscles and bones. As we age, our bones tend to lose calcium and weaken. This process, called osteoporosis, affects women more than men. There is no cure, but a diet rich in vitamin D, calcium and protein can help to prevent or stop the problem. Be sure to eat lots of dark green, leafy vegetables like Swiss chard and

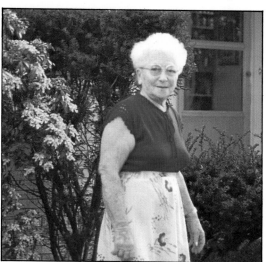

If you are living alone, it's important to make sure you keep up your interest in food, as it's all too easy to neglect your dietary needs. This can have particularly serious consequences as you grow older, and naturally become vulnerable to injury or infection.

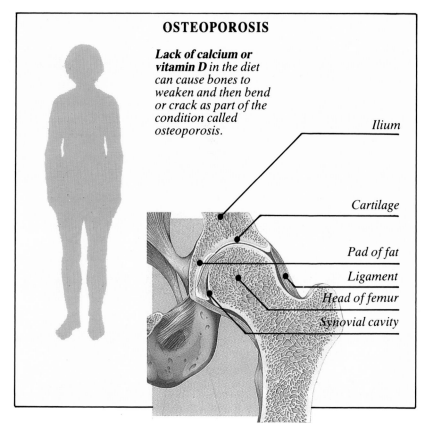

OSTEOPOROSIS

Lack of calcium or vitamin D in the diet can cause bones to weaken and then bend or crack as part of the condition called osteoporosis.

Ilium

Cartilage

Pad of fat

Ligament

Head of femur

Synovial cavity

Chinese bok choy, and talk to your doctor about taking a vitamin supplement.

Tiredness caused by inadequate nourishment contributes to the apathy many elderly people feel. The social aspect of eating is important to all of us, particularly in these circumstances. Try to arrange social events involving meals. Share in the purchasing and preparation of the food with friends. Have a pot-luck dinner, where every guest brings a prepared dish to add to the feast. Take charge and assign certain food groups to people to prevent a glut of cakes and pies or an absence of fruits and salads.

If you have a favorite but complicated dish, try making a large batch. Then you can divide up the dish into smaller portions, store it in your freezer, and be able to enjoy it for a few weeks. Just because you may be alone, there's no reason to deprive yourself of the things you enjoy! Make that big, juicy turkey and afterward you can continue to dine on the big bird as fixings for sandwiches, salads, or even as a filling for a turkey and vegetable pie!

SAVING CALORIES

Since none of us wants to spend the rest of our life eating little more than a bowl of brown rice and fruits, it's important that we get into the habit of looking for ways to diversify the diet. We can still continue to eat delicious meals and keep on a healthy regimen, if we learn to save calories. By "saving calories" we don't mean that you starve on Tuesday so that you can double up on Wednesday! Saving calories means substituting a low-calorie ingredient for a more fattening and unhealthy one.

For example, many of us are in the habit of munching pretzels and potato chips while watching television. Few of us have the nerve to read the label on the snack packages. If we did, we'd see all sorts of unhealthy ingredients, including saturated fats and salt. So next time you get the urge to munch, save a few calories. Instead of a one-ounce bag of potato chips, eat a cup of plain popcorn. Besides adding fiber to your diet, this switch from potato chips to popcorn saves you 150 calories.

Since many of us suffer from a sweet tooth, we'd better come up with a substitute for those unhealthy sugary treats. Surprisingly, there's a new product at your supermarket — one that's been a mainstay in health-food stores for years — rice cakes. The next time you're about to reach for the cookie jar, try a low-calorie rice cake instead. Rice cakes are made only with brown rice — no additives, no sugar. In fact, most have little or no sodium. If you haven't tasted these treats, you'll never believe how sweet they seem. The bonding process that forms the cakes turns the brown rice into a satisfying delight, for only 35 calories!

You're at the office picnic and while everyone else is huddling around the potato salad and hamburgers, you look for something that's more in tune with your new health awareness. Since it's not the potato in the potato salad that's fattening (it's the mayonnaise), try eating the vegetables themselves. You save about 150 calories by eating one cup of raw vegetables instead of half a cup of potato salad.

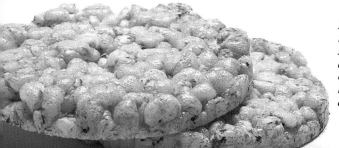

Rice cakes *make perfect snacks. They are low in calories, healthy and delicious.*

CALORIE-CUTTING TIPS

● There are a number of things you can do to cut calories and still eat properly. For example, all of us have favorite foods. The problem is that putting a platter of your favorite food in front of your place at the table can be dieting suicide. So what can you do? Short of sitting on your hands as everybody else digs in, one solution calls for you to just take a smaller portion.

● Reducing the size of the portions of your food cuts calories. Half of anything is quite simply . . . half of anything. If you simply cannot resist seconds, you can take a little more. The end result is you've still eaten just one portion instead of gorging.

● Another calorie-cutter involves understanding the mechanisms behind the appestat, the hunger control center in the brain. It takes about 20 minutes for your brain to realize that food has entered your stomach. Many overweight people eat so quickly that the brain doesn't have time to react to the food. They continue eating and then suddenly feel bloated. The solution? Eat slowly. Allow the food to control your appetite. Try counting as you chew, instead of gulping it down. Along those lines, try eating a piece of whole-wheat bread about 20 minutes before meal time. This will put your ravenous appetite under control even before you sit down at the table. The less hungry you feel, the less likely you are to overeat!

● Since we now know that saturated fats are unhealthy, and add calories, you should roast, broil, bake, poach, or steam your food rather than frying.
 Another high-calorie product is alcohol. One fluid ounce of alcohol contains about 65 calories. Drinking at cocktail parties can put on the pounds. Try instead some white wine mixed with club soda. Not only will you cut down on the calories, but you'll reduce your alcohol consumption.

● Even though chicken and turkey are high protein sources, the skin of these birds is high in fat. In fact, the skin is probably higher in calories than the meat. Try removing the skin of poultry and fish. Ideally, you should remove this skin before cooking. However, unless you are deft with a knife this can be quite difficult. But after the chicken or fish is cooked, you can peel off the skin and peel off those pounds!

SALAD STAPLES

Fresh vegetables should look as good as they taste and can be used together in hundreds of imaginative ways to produce exciting salads. Some of the more interesting lettuces include:

- endive which has a sharp bitter flavor.
- chicory which has a more delicate bitter flavor.
- pak-choi is a Chinese vegetable now widely cultivated. It is recognizable by its chalk-white stalks.
- Chinese cabbage with a taste that is a cross between those of cabbage and celery.
- watercress with a delicate peppery taste.
- oakleaf lettuce which is an unusual loose-headed lettuce.
- spinach which is a very versatile although delicate vegetable.
- raddichio which is available in a variety of different colors.
- iceberg lettuce with its super crisp leaves and flavorful hearts.
- romaine lettuce which is characterized by its strong sharp taste.

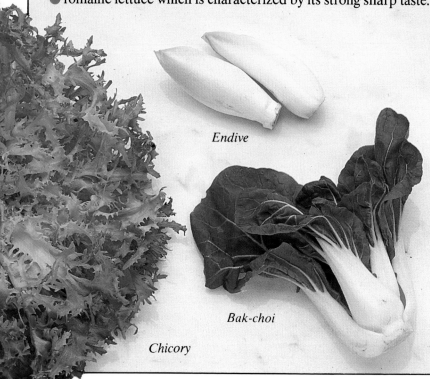

Endive

Bak-choi

Chicory

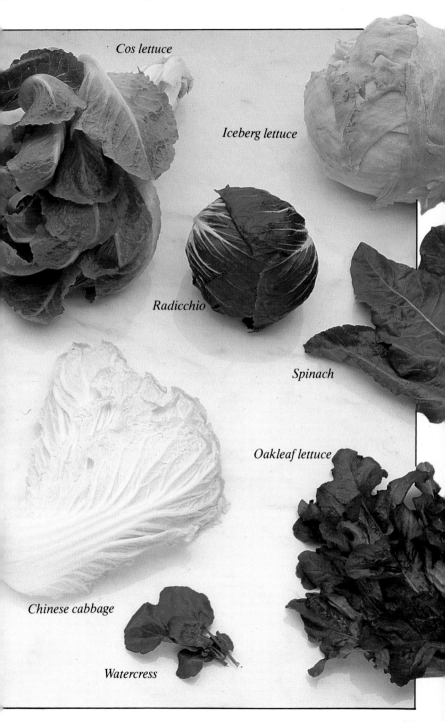

Cos lettuce

Iceberg lettuce

Radicchio

Spinach

Oakleaf lettuce

Chinese cabbage

Watercress

KEEPING SLIM OVER THE WEEKEND

You've made it through the week! Exercising, dieting, and feeling pretty good about yourself, have made it a good one. Friday night rolls around and the "new you" is about ready to socialize. Party-hopping, going out to dinner, enjoying a nice leisurely brunch are all ways to sabotage your diet. Here are a few tips to help you keep going through the weekend:

● If you're going to do any drinking, keep away from the whiskey sours, beer, eggnogs and creamy concoctions. Instead, go with lower-calorie white wines, vodka, and gin. By choosing the right alcohol, you can save 500 calories a night!

● If you're entertaining at your home, take advantage of the situation by preparing a number of low-calorie alternatives to the average party fare. Since only a bad hostess forces her guests to eat low-calorie food, give them the choice. Put some celery and carrot sticks next to the snack foods.

● Try to eat a little something before going out. If you hit a party simply starving for food, you're going to destroy your diet. Another suggestion is to make sure you do not stand around the food table. Sometimes just being around the food is enough of a temptation for you to snack. Soon you'll be snacking your way to a larger dress size.

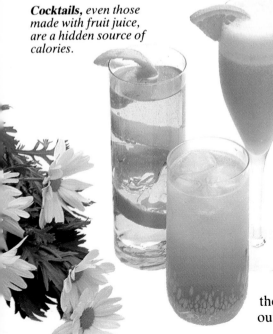

Cocktails, even those made with fruit juice, are a hidden source of calories.

● Just because it's the weekend, don't ignore your exercises. Many people just want to relax and enjoy their two days. Remember that during the week, you're burning up calories at work by being active. On weekends without the exercise of work, you'll have to try harder to keep in shape. If you're not the type to exercise, then increase the housework schedule. Get out there and mow the lawn.

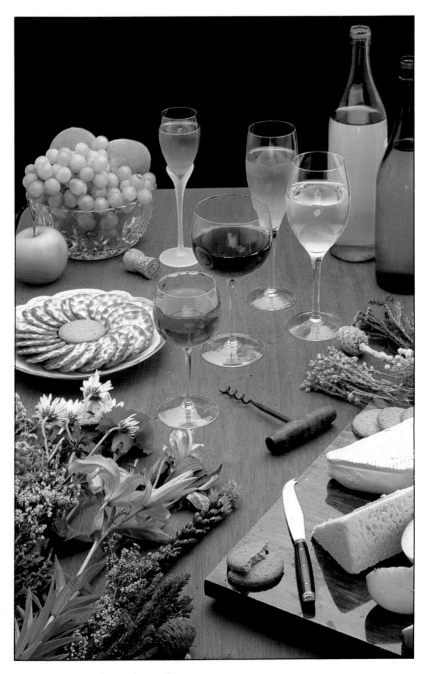

Buffet-style parties *make it all too easy to nibble all evening long.*

THE SALAD BAR SURVIVAL GUIDE

As part of the general increase in health awareness around the country, many restaurants now have salad bars. Yet despite the advantage of being able to select your own food, many of us would be better off, calorie-wise, by ordering right off the menu! Like any other source of food, the salad bar has its benefits and drawbacks.

You grab your plate, saunter over to the bar and begin piling on the chickpeas, bacon bits, cheese, chicken salad and a heaping helping of creamy dressing. Congratulations! You have just piled up what could amount to over 2,500 calories, the target amount for the entire day! But don't despair, here are a few tips on salad bar survival:

● Stay away from the creamy dressings, marinated salads and fattening toppings. These garnishes are calorie-ladden and salad bar enemies.

● Since most of the dressings are loaded with fat, additives, preservatives, and artificial flavorings, try using a little lemon juice or yogurt instead.

● Fresh vegetables are always a better alternative to prepared salads such as egg or tuna. Most restaurants use mayonnaise to prepare these salads. Mayonnaise is high in calories and cholesterol.

NON-FATTENING SALAD DRESSINGS

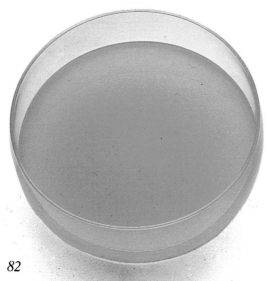

MODERN VINAIGRETTE

MAKES 1 CUP
2 tbsp wine vinegar
1 tbsp lemon juice
1 tbsp mustard
¼ tsp salt
⅛ tsp black pepper
¾ cup olive oil

Put vinegar, lemon juice, mustard, salt and pepper in a jar with a lid and shake until salt dissolves. Add olive oil and shake well before serving.

Here are some sampling of typical salad bar items and their calorie content. Remember these are rough estimates and should be taken, pardon the expression, with a grain of salt.

Food	Amount	Calories
lettuce	1 cup	10
beets	½ cup	26
avocado	medium	190
carrots	½ cup	25
chickpeas	½ cup	360
onion	½ cup	38
mushrooms	½ cup	10
red cabbage	½ cup	12
red kidney beans	½ cup	108
tomato	½ cup	20
chicken salad	1 scoop	200
American cheese	1 ounce	102
Cheddar cheese	1 ounce	70
bacon bits	1 ounce	188
raisins	1 ounce	83
chow mein noodles	1 ounce	139
Italian dressing	1 tablespoon	83
Yogurt dressing	1 tablespoon	9

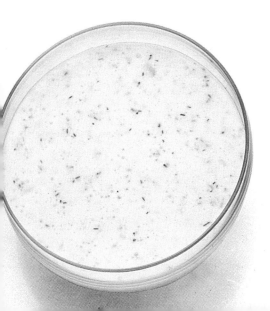

BUTTERMILK DRESSING

MAKES 1 CUP
½ cup buttermilk
2 tbsp olive oil
1 tbsp finely chopped onion
3 tbsp lemon juice
1 tsp dried dill
¼ tsp salt

Put all ingredients in a blender and blend well or whisk well by hand before serving.

THE FAST FOOD BLITZ

In today's modern world you may not be able to escape the clutches of the fast food restaurant. With most foods prepared in advance and containing the inevitable secret sauce, eating at a fast food restaurant can be very upsetting to your health-conscious style of eating.

However, if you learn to be selective, some of these foods have the convenience of being fast and fresh. Remember to watch your calories, because if you do it right, you'll get the dieting break you deserve.

Here is the caloric analysis for some fast foods from the leading chains:

McDonald's	calories
Hamburger, plain	255
Cheeseburger	307
Big Mac	563
Fries, regular	220
Filet-o-Fish	432
Chicken McNuggets	330
Quarter pounder	424
Vanilla shake	352
Apple pie	253
Egg McMuffin	340

Kentucky Fried Chicken	calories
Original recipe:	
wing	136
breast	199
drumstick	177
thigh	257
Extra Crispy recipe:	
wing	201
breast	286
drumstick	255
thigh	343
Mashed potatoes	64
Fries	184

Burger King	
Cheeseburger	350
Whopper	630
Double Beef Whopper	850
Fries	210
Onion rings	270
Hamburger	290
Whopper with cheese	740
Apple pie	240

Taco Bell	
Bean burrito	343
Bellbeefer with cheese	278
Pintos 'n' Cheese	168
Tostada	179
Burrito Supreme	457
Taco	186

In response to recent consumer requests, most fast food chains now have booklets available detailing the nutritional analysis of their products. If not displayed on the counter, ask the manager for a copy.

A hamburger may not affect your diet, but add catsup, french fries and mass-produced apple pie, and you will be piling up the calories without satisfying your nutritional requirements.

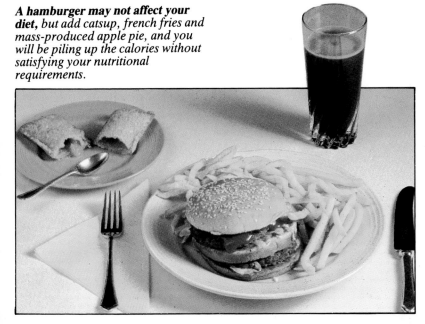

THE DINING OUT GUIDE

Just because you're on a diet doesn't mean you can't eat out at a fine restaurant once in a while. In fact, learning how to eat out should be a part of your new diet. This will help when you begin concentrating on maintaining the new, thinner you!

Here are a few hints on how to cope with the dinner:

● **TAKE YOUR TIME AND READ THE MENU CAREFULLY.** You're not in any rush. You've taken the time the past few weeks to shed those pounds; let's not put them back at one meal. Look for those dishes such as fish or poultry that are good for you and low in calories. Make sure that they'll be prepared in a low-fat manner, such as broiling or baking. Keep away from dishes that are fried or breaded. You also should not order anything stuffed, because that's exactly what you don't want to become!

● **EAT SLOWLY AND DON'T CLEAN THE PLATE.** If you eat slowly, not only will you be able to enjoy the texture and aroma of the food, but you'll be giving the appetite control mechanism in your brain time to catch up with your stomach. Also, despite your mother's warnings about cleaning your plate or no dessert, don't eat everything. Eat until you are satisfied and then, if you'd like, ask the waiter to wrap the remainder up for you to take away.

● **BE CREATIVE.** The menu is arranged in the customary start-to-finish manner, but be creative with your selections. If you want an appetizer and all that's offered are fattening selections, look to the dessert menu and select some fresh fruit.

● **WATCH OUT FOR HIDDEN CALORIES.** Here they come again, those calorie commandos hiding in your drink or salad dressing. Ambush those calories by drinking white wine with club soda and asking the waiter for a non-creamy salad dressing on the side. Then you become the general of your dinner and send those hidden calories away from your waistline!

Smaller portions are no longer thought of as being "mean" as more people become conscious of the need for healthy eating habits.

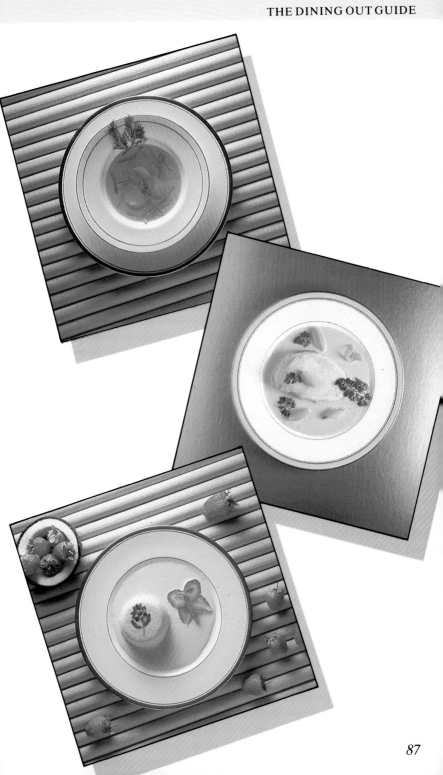

LOSING THOSE LAST FEW POUNDS

You've stuck to your diet plans and kept exercising, but those last few pounds just won't come off. It might be that your body is at its limit. In that case, you might consider changing to a maintainence diet and keep your exercises going. But if you are thoroughly convinced that those few pounds just have to go, here are some tips and words of encouragement.

● When you sit down to eat, don't let anything distract you. As silly as it sounds, you must concentrate on eating and nothing else. Watching television or reading will prevent you from dealing with what may be an eating problem — eating too quickly. Remember, the faster you eat, the more food you'll consume before your hunger eases. Too many of us shovel in the food while we watch television, never really knowing how much we've eaten until the fork hits the bottom of the pan.

● Try to increase your level and amount of exercise slightly. It might be that your current exercise program, although perfect for a maintainence regimen, needs a little more zip to shed those remaining pounds.

Although packed with goodness, dried fruits are a concentrated source of energy. By all means incorporate them into your diet — topped perhaps with some low-fat yogurt — but be wary of overindulging.

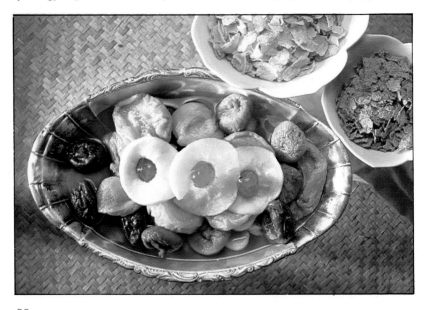

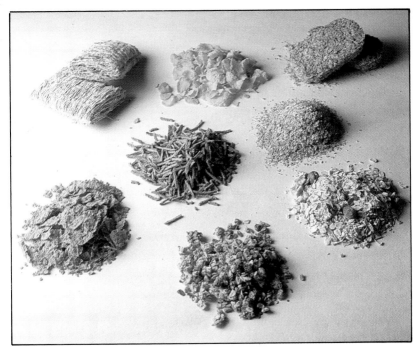

Don't be tempted to shed those remaining pounds by skipping breakfast. *Without an energy boost first thing you will become sluggish and less mentally alert as the morning wears on and also more* *prone to snack on unsuitable foods. If cereal (top) is your preferred choice, go for one with a minimum of added salt and sugar and a high fiber content.*

● Don't try to cheat your system by skipping breakfast. You need that energy surge in the morning. Besides, the body's metabolism burns food up quicker early in the day.

● As crazy as it sounds, brush your teeth more often. You'll be less likely to eat after brushing your teeth nice and white.

● Try to keep busy at work and at home. Working on projects other than these last few pounds will take your mind off food and might just be the trick.

● You might try increasing the fiber in your diet. Fiber helps to fill you up while helping to clean the intestines.

● If all else fails, learn to live with the few extra pounds. You've probably underestimated the proper weight for your body. Remember, those charts of ideal weights are approximate. We all have different body types and daily requirements. Besides, nobody is going to take a look at the new, thinner you and say, "Hey, I think you could still lose a pound."

LOW-CALORIE LUNCHES

Between your energy-boosting breakfast and carefully prepared dinner comes lunch. Since most of us have only a limited time to eat lunch, and many of us eat lunch out, the meal is often neglected — we either skip lunch altogether, or eat fast food or deli sandwiches, both loaded with calories. Eating a good, healthy lunch will leave you feeling satisfied and help you get through the rest of the working day. And you'll be less ravenous when you get home, so you'll want to eat less at dinner.

A good tip for a low-calorie lunch is to make open-faced sandwiches using healthy ingredients. You'll feel like you're getting more to eat. For example, try an open-face turkey sandwich, using two ounces sliced turkey on whole-wheat bread. Season it with freshly ground black pepper and pile on all the lettuce leaves and tomato slices you want. It's low in calories and delicious!

Here's a great recipe for a favorite lunchtime standby:

TUNA SALAD

1 6½ ounce can water-packed tuna
⅓ cup unflavored low-fat yogurt
1 teaspoon prepared mustard
greshly ground black pepper to taste
¼ cup finely chopped onion
¼ cup chopped celery

Drain the liquid from the tuna. Combine all the ingredients in a bowl and mix well. Serve on whole-grain bread with lettuce leaves and tomato slices.

As the tuna salad recipe shows, by being creative you can have a low-calorie lunch and enjoy it, too. You can take any of your favorite luncheon treats and take out the fattening parts. For example, the tuna salad recipe here substitutes yogurt for the traditional mayonnaise.

Another way to cut calories at lunch time is to keep away from the breads. Most salads are delicious as is; you won't miss the taste or the calories from the bread. And speaking of sandwiches, remember that most processed meats and cheese are loaded with salt, additives and calories.

SALSA
(MEXICAN HOT SAUCE)

MAKES 2½ CUPS
CALORIES PER SERVING: 16

3 large, ripe tomatoes
1 onion, finely chopped
1 tablespoon olive oil
2 tablespoons wine vinegar
½ to ¾ long green chili pepper, seeded and finely chopped
2 tablespoons chopped fresh coriander or fresh parsley

● Blanch the tomatoes by placing them in a large pot of boiling water for about 10 seconds. Drain the tomatoes. When they are cool enough to handle, peel with a small, sharp knife. Seed and chop the tomatoes.

● Combine the tomatoes and onion in a large bowl. Add the oil and vinegar and mix well. Add green chili to taste, beginning with half the chili pepper.

● Sprinkle with the fresh coriander or parsley.

● Simmer gently for 10 minutes to blend the flavors.

● Serve hot or cold, garnished with the watercress sprigs.

WATERCRESS AND POTATO SOUP

SERVES 6
CALORIES PER SERVING: 145

1½ tablespoons unsalted butter
3 whole scallions, minced
1 carrot, peeled and grated
3½ cups water
3 large Idaho potatoes, peeled and cut
into ½-inch slices
1 cup chopped watercress, tough stems removed
½ cup unflavored low-fat yogurt
½ cup low-fat milk
freshly ground black pepper
6 watercress sprigs

● Melt the butter in a large, heavy pot over low heat. Add the scallions and carrot. Cover the pot and cook until the vegetables are very soft, about 5 to 8 minutes.

● Add the potatoes and water to the pot. Cover, raise heat to medium, and cook until the potatoes are tender, about 20 minutes.

● Puree the contents of the pot in batches in a blender or food processor. Return the mixture to the pot and stir in the watercress, yogurt, milk, and black pepper to taste. To make the soup by hand, remove the vegetables from the liquid with a slotted spoon. Put them in a small bowl and mash them. Return the mashed vegetables to the soup and blend well. Add the remaining ingredients.

DILLED CUCUMBER SALAD

SERVES 6
CALORIES PER SERVING: 30

2 large cucumbers, peeled and thinly sliced
3 whole scallions, thinly sliced
2 tablespoons sugar
2 tablespoons white vinegar
4 tablespoons water
¼ teaspoon coarsely ground black pepper
¼ cup chopped fresh dill

● Put the cucumber slices between sheets of paper towel. With your hands, squeeze as much liquid from the slices as possible.

● Put the cucumbers and scallions into a serving bowl.

● In a small bowl, dissolve the sugar in the vinegar. Add the water and black pepper and mix well. Pour the mixture over the cucumbers and onions and mix well. Let the salad stand at room temperature for 10 minutes to blend the flavors. Sprinkle with the chopped dill and serve.

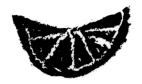

RECIPES FOR HEALTHY EATERS

It's really very easy to cook healthy, satisfying meals for your family. Just remember the basic food groups and use your imagination to modify your favorite dishes or create new ones. Some excellent cookbooks with a whole-foods approach are available at any library or bookstore. Check them out for ideas, and try some of the easy-to-prepare dishes suggested here.

POTATO TOPPER

MAKES 1 CUP
CALORIES PER TABLESPOON: 10

1 cup low-fat cottage cheese
1 tablespoon skim milk
2 teaspoons lemon juice
chopped scallions or parsley for garnish

● Combine the cottage cheese, skim milk, and lemon juice in a bowl or blender. Mix or blend thoroughly until the mixture is smooth and creamy. Chill.
● Serve over baked or boiled potatoes. Garnish with chopped scallions or parsley.

LOW-CALORIE FRENCH DRESSING

MAKES 1 CUP
CALORIES PER TABLESPOON: 10

1½ tablespoons cornstarch
2 tablespoons sugar
1 cup water
¼ cup white vinegar
½ teaspoon dry mustard
½ teaspoon paprika
⅛ teaspoon onion powder
⅛ teaspoon garlic powder

● Combine the cornstarch and sugar in a saucepan. Stir in the water.
● Cook over low heat, stirring constantly, until the mixture thickens.
● Remove the saucepan from the heat and let the mixture cool slightly. Add the remaining ingredients and mix thoroughly. Chill.

LEMON-BAKED CHICKEN

SERVES 4
CALORIES PER SERVING: 135

3 tablespoons lemon juice
2 tablespoons water
¼ teaspoon onion powder
¼ teaspoon dried marjoram leaves
⅛ teaspoon paprika
4 skinless chicken breasts
parsley sprigs for garnish

● Preheat the oven to 350°F.
● Combine the lemon juice, water,

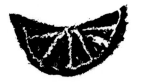

onion powder, marjoram and paprika in a small bowl. Mix well.

● Arrange the chicken breasts in a shallow baking dish. Pour the lemon-juice mixture over the breasts.

● Bake for 50 minutes, or until the breasts are tender, basting occasionally.

● Garnish with parsley sprigs and serve with rice.

● Add the vegetables to the skillet and cook, stirring constantly, until the vegetables are tender but still crisp.

● Stir the cornstarch mixture and add it to the skillet. Stir well and continue to cook until the sauce thickens. Serve over rice.

BEEF WITH CHINESE-STYLE VEGETABLES

SERVES 4
CALORIES PER SERVING: 190

1 pound lean, boneless beef round steak
2 teaspoons vegetable oil
2/3 cup green beans, thinly julienned
2/3 cup carrots, thinly julienned
2/3 cup peeled turnips, thinly julienned
2/3 cup Chinese or green cabbage, thinly julienned
4 teaspoons cornstarch
1/2 teaspoon ground ginger
1/8 teaspoon garlic powder
1 tablespoon soy sauce
1/3 cup water

● Trim any visible fat from the beef. Slice the beef across the grain into thin strips about 1/8-inch wide and 3 inches long. (This is easier to do if the meat is partially frozen.)

● In a small bowl combine the cornstarch, ginger, garlic, soy sauce and water. Mix well and set aside.

● Heat the oil in a large skillet over high heat. Add the beef strips and cook, stirring constantly, until the beef loses its redness, about 2 to 3 minutes.

POTATO SALAD WITH LOW-CALORIE DRESSING

SERVES 8
CALORIES PER SERVING: 175

6 medium-sized russet potatoes
1 1/2 green peppers, chopped
1 1/2 sweet red peppers, chopped
4 whole scallions, chopped
1 cup unflavored low-fat yogurt
1/2 cup salt-free Dijon-style mustard
1/4 cup red wine vinegar
freshly ground black pepper

● Put the potatoes into a large saucepan. Add water to cover and boil for 25 minutes, or until the potatoes can just be easily pierced with a fork. Immediately drain the potatoes and rinse under cold water.

● Peel and slice the potatoes while they are still warm. Put slices into a serving bowl.

● In a small bowl, combine the green and red peppers, scallions, yogurt, mustard, vinegar, and black pepper. Whisk well to blend. Pour the dressing over the warm, sliced potatoes and mix gently but well. The warm potatoes will absorb the flavors of the dressing. Serve at room temperature.

SPAGHETTI PRIMAVERA

SERVES 4
CALORIES PER SERVING: 612

2 tablespoons olive oil
2 tablespoons unsalted butter
2 garlic cloves, minced
3½ cups young zucchini
or summer squash, cut into ¼-inch
rounds
1½ cups whole leeks, cut into 2-inch
pieces
2 cups stemmed whole cherry
tomatoes
2 cups thin asparagus, cut into 2-inch
pieces
2 tablespoons lemon juice
2 tablespoons red wine (optional)
1 cup spinach, torn into 2-inch pieces
3 tablespoons chopped fresh basil
2 tablespoons chopped fresh parsley
freshly ground black pepper
1 pound very thin spaghetti

● Heat the oil and butter in a large, heavy skillet. Add the garlic, zucchini, leeks, cherry tomatoes and asparagus and sauté over medium heat for 7 minutes, or until the asparagus is tender. Add the lemon juice and red wine. Cook about 1½ minutes. Add the spinach, basil, parsley, and black pepper to taste. Mix well. Remove the skillet from the heat and cover.
● Cook the spaghetti. When done, drain well and put into a large serving bowl. Add the vegetable mixture and toss gently. Serve warm or at room temperature.

POACHED FISH WITH ALMONDS

SERVES 4
CALORIES PER SERVING: 358

4 tablespoons unsalted butter
⅔ cup slivered almonds
¼ cup white wine
¼ cup lemon juice
½ cup water
¼ teaspoon white pepper
1½ pounds fish fillets

● Melt the butter in a large heavy skillet. Add the almonds and sauté, stirring frequently, until they begin to turn golden. Remove the almonds with a slotted spoon and drain on paper towels. Set aside.
● Add the wine, lemon juice, water and white pepper to the skillet. Stir well and bring to a simmer. Add the fish fillets and spoon the sauce over them.
● Cover the skillet and gently poach the fillets until the fish flakes easily with a fork, about 7 to 8 minutes.
● Place the fish on a serving platter. Spoon the sauce over the fillets and sprinkle with the almonds. Serve immediately.

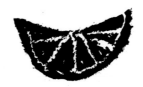

INDEX

Page numbers in *italic* refer to the illustrations and captions